CHINESE MEDICINE CURES

DEPRESSION

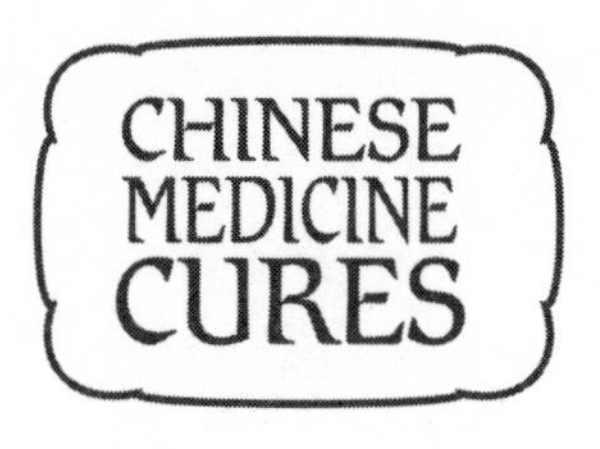

DEPRESSION

BOB FLAWS AND ROSA N. SCHYNER

Adapted for the UK by Sylvia Schroer

foulsham
LONDON • NEW YORK • TORONTO • SYDNEY

foulsham
The Publishing House, Bennetts Close,
Cippenham, Berkshire SL1 5AP, England

ISBN 0-572-02577-7

Neither the editors of W. Foulsham and Co. Ltd nor the author nor the publisher take responsibility for any possible consequences from any treatment, procedure, test, exercise, action or application of medication or preparation by any person reading or following the information in this book. The publication of this book does not constitute the practice of medicine, and this book does not attempt to replace your doctor. The author and publisher advise the reader to check with a doctor before administering any medication or undertaking any course of treatment or exercise.

Printed in Great Britain by St. Edmundsbury Press, Bury St. Edmunds, Suffolk

CONTENTS

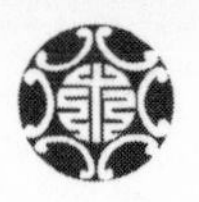

PREFACE

Depression seems to be epidemic in our society. Every day, we meet people who are currently on antidepressants. The discovery of a new line of medications, such as Zoloft and Prozac, has made antidepressants easily administered, widely used and almost certainly over-prescribed. The rapidly growing demands of our modern lifestyles submit us to very high levels of physical and emotional stress. We may find ourselves depleted of inner resources, struggling to catch up.

Depression affects people's lives in profound ways. It touches every aspect of the human experience – our physical well-being, our relationships with our loved ones, our work, our creativity, our spirituality. Depression can paralyse and alienate us, making us strangers to ourselves and to the world we inhabit.

As an acupuncturist and practitioner of Chinese medicine involved in research funded in the USA by the National Institutes of Health (NIH), I have had the opportunity to assist numerous people suffering from depression. I have seen Chinese medicine help transform hopelessness into possibility, helplessness into courage, anxiety into calmness. With the help of Bob Flaws, I have written this book as a comprehensive guide for laypeople to the treatment of depression with Chinese medicine. It presents an overview of the fundamental principles that underlie the theory and practice of acupuncture and Chinese herbal medicine. It instructs the reader on preventive techniques and numerous home remedies, and provides information on how to create an individual regime.

We live in a society accustomed to avoiding pain, that refuses delayed gratification and resists any change that requires effort. The idea of altering our mood and escaping the complexity of a depressive episode quickly and effortlessly is quite appealing. Our tendency to reduce biological and psychological processes to mechanistic interactions reinforces the treatment of depression as a linear event. If there is a deficit of neurotransmitters such as serotonin, then making more serotonin available should resolve depression. There is no doubt that antidepressants are sometimes indispensable and may be life-saving for many people. However, these drugs fail to address the more complex chain of interactions, both biological and psychological, that typically contribute to depression.

Currently, there is a new wave of enthusiasm for replacing antidepressant drugs with botanical extracts, for example, St John's wort *(Hypericum perforatum)*. St. John's wort has been widely tested in Europe in the treatment of mild to moderate depression. While this natural approach may have clear advantages over conventional drugs (it has no known side-effects!), it fails to treat the person as a whole and still approaches depression as an entity separate from the person.

Chinese medicine offers an alternative and complementary approach to the understanding and treatment of depression. It aims to integrate body and mind. It is free of side-effects and can empower the person to make changes in their life. With this book, we hope to make the wealth of information on the Chinese medical treatment of this devastating disease widely available to readers in the West. We also hope that it contributes to eradicating the stigma associated with psychological distress and mental illness in general.

Rosa N. Schnyer

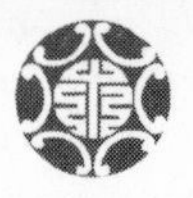

INTRODUCTION

Joan was feeling increasingly irritable and frustrated. She often wanted to hide and not see people and she had no desire to do anything at all. She had lost interest in life and felt apathetic. She was tired all the time and even spent long periods of time just staring at the wall. Though she was always exhausted, she also felt restless and anxious. She fidgeted constantly whilst sitting at her desk trying to do her job, which she hated. She had gained quite a bit of weight because she always felt hungry. Food calmed her down, but it also made her sluggish and bloated. Often she would burst out crying over minor things and had difficulty sleeping through the night. Her dreams were vivid and disturbing.

If this story sounds familiar, this book may help you overcome the cycle of depression. Practitioners of Chinese medicine have treated the symptoms of depression safely and effectively for centuries

This book is a layperson's guide to the diagnosis and treatment of depression. In it, you will learn the Chinese medical perspective on what causes depression and what you can do about it. It is our hope that you will be able to recognise yourself and your symptoms in these pages. If you can see yourself in the signs and symptoms we discuss in this book, we feel confident that we will be able to share with you a number of self-help techniques that can minimise your discomfort. One of us has been a professional practitioner of Chinese medicine for over 10 years and has helped many Western patients cure, relieve or manage their depression. No system of medicine can cure every disease, but when it comes to depression Chinese medicine is a valuable alternative. Not only is Chinese medicine very effective for curing or at least reducing the symptoms of depression, but if you follow the advice presented in this book you can also help prevent the recurrence of depressive episodes. Long-term, chronic depression and depression complicated by other factors can also be addressed by Chinese medicine. Chinese medicine may not totally eradicate these more complicated and recalcitrant types of depression, but it can certainly help alleviate some of the symptoms and help with management of the condition.

WHAT IS DEPRESSION?

Depression is a pervasive, low mood disorder that may affect every aspect of normal functioning. It is associated with other symptoms including poor sleep, irritability, anxiety, appetite and weight disturbances, loss of libido, low energy, poor concentration, obsessive/compulsive thoughts, low self-esteem and in more severe cases thoughts of suicide. According to the *British Medical Journal* (Vol 315 (7099), pp 43–6, 5 July 1997) one in 20 visits to a family doctor is connected with depression. Depression can be associated with other psychiatric illnesses, such as schizophrenia or manic depression, which also has an elated phase. It can be a reaction to external events, in which case it is known as reactive or exogenous depression, or it can occur with no apparent or obvious trigger, in which case it is known as endogenous depression. The majority of people who suffer from depression also suffer from anxiety. As an illness, depression may be seen on a continuum, from moderate or mild through to severe depression, which might occur with psychotic features such as delusions or hallucinations. Should depression continue for several years or more, it is known as chronic depression. Some depression may also be associated with seasonal change, and this is known as Seasonal Affective Disorder (SAD). Depression may sometimes be referred to as dysthymia, or in the case of manic depression as cyclothymia. Another term for mild depression is melancholia. In some cases, depression may be associated with a chronic illness such as anorexia, multiple sclerosis or rheumatoid arthritis, in which case it may be called secondary dysthymia.

A milder yet more prevalent form of depression

A recent study in the USA headed by Dr Louis Judd, former director of the National Institutes of Mental Health, found that many people who do not meet the current diagnostic criteria for depression nevertheless suffer from a real impairment due to one or more symptoms of this illness. Often such sufferers lack the symptoms of a depressed mood. This milder depression is four times more prevalent than clinical depression. The three most common symptoms reported in this case are fatigue, sleep disturbance and thoughts of death. Dr Judd calls this condition 'subsyndromal symptomatic depression'.[1] This study highlights the fact that there are many people suffering from some, albeit less severe, aspects of depressive illness.

CAUSES OF DEPRESSION

For years Western clinicians and researchers have debated whether the causes of depression are essentially biological and related to brain chemistry or more psychological in nature. This mind/body debate is common to all Western sciences. There may also be genetic factors involved, particularly with regard to manic depression, or bipolar disorder.

HOW WESTERN MEDICINE TREATS DEPRESSION

The treatment of depression in Western medicine relates to the mind/body debate previously mentioned. The two main

---

[1] Michal, Norden J, *Beyond Prozac*, HarperCollins Publishers Inc., NY, 1995.

treatment approaches involve medication or psychotherapy and sometimes a combination of both.

Pharmacotherapy means the administration of internal medicines. It is based on the biological perspective of depression and it basically involves the prescription of antidepressants. The very latest medications to be used in the UK are seratonin noradrenaline re-uptake inhibitors (SNRIs), an example of which is Venlafixine. Most frequently prescribed nowadays are the selective seratonin re-uptake inhibitors (SSRIs), such as Prozac, Seroxat and Lustral. The next most commonly used antidepressants are the tricyclic antidepressants (TCAs), which include Imipramine, Amitriptyline, Dothiepin and Lofepramine. Finally, monoamine oxidase inhibitors (MAOIs), which include Nardil, are the least frequently prescribed.

Unfortunately, antidepressants have a wide range of side-effects. For example, if MAOIs are taken in combination with a diet that includes chocolate, oranges, cheese and other foods that contain large amounts of tyramine, they can cause high blood pressure. The side-effects caused by the tricyclics are not as dangerous as this, but they are quite unpleasant none the less. These include drowsiness, blurred vision, constipation and a dry mouth. The SSRIs, such as Prozac, can cause headache, anxiety, upset stomach and decreased libido or sexual desire. They can also cause agitation, violence and thoughts of suicide in a small number of people.

The psychotherapeutic treatment of depression includes three main approaches: psychodynamic, humanistic–existential and cognitive–behavioural. Each of these approaches emphasises a different theory of the causation of depression. It is not within the scope of this book to go more deeply into these treatment approaches, but further information is included in the Bibliography (see pages 167–72). In terms of psychotherapy, Cognitive Behavioural Therapy (CBT) is considered one of the most effective approaches to the treatment of depression. The current medical standard care combines the use of antidepressants with short-term psychotherapy.

Both the pharmacological and psychotherapeutic approaches alleviate depression in 50–70 per cent of people who complete treatment, but a significant number of people terminate therapy prior to its completion. Depression tends to be a chronic disorder and is likely to recur, even when it is successfully treated with either Western drugs or psychotherapy. There is a general consensus among those who treat depression that some form of continued maintenance treatment is necessary after initial recovery has occurred.

Chinese medicine offers safe, effective, low-cost alternatives for the treatment of depression that have been used in Asia for thousands of years. Chinese medicine not only has a good record of success, but with the correct treatment it also has few side-effects. It can be preventive and it addresses both the body and mind. In fact, as we will see below, there is no division between the body and mind in Chinese medicine. Additionally, Chinese medicine empowers patients to make changes in their lives and participate in their own health recuperation and maintenance.

EAST IS EAST AND WEST IS WEST

In order to understand and make sense of the rest of this book on Chinese medicine and depression, it is important to understand that Chinese medicine is a distinct and separate system of medical thought and practice from modern Western medicine. This means shifting models of reality when it comes to thinking about Chinese medicine. It has taken the Chinese more than 2,000 years to develop this medical system. In fact, Chinese medicine is the oldest continually practised, literate system of medicine in the world. It is best to approach Chinese medicine on its own terms, rather than trying to explain it according to Western medical science.

Most people reading this book will have some basic knowledge of biology. Whether we recognise it or not, most of us Westerners think of what we learned about the human body at school as the one true description of reality, not just one possible description. If Chinese medicine is to make any sense to Westerners at all, we need to accept that there may be other valid descriptions of the human body, its functions, health and disease. In grappling with this fundamentally important issue, it is useful to think about the concepts of a map and the terrain it describes.

If we take the United Kingdom as an example, we can have numerous different maps of this country's land mass. One map might show population. Another might show per capita incomes. Another might show geographical features or simply be a road map. We could also show county boundaries. In fact, there could be an infinite number of potentially different maps of the United Kingdom depending on what one was trying to show and do. As long as the map is based on accurate information and has been created with self-consistent logic, then one map is not necessarily more correct than another. The important thing is to use the right map for what you are trying to do. If you wanted to drive from London to Glasgow for example, a road map is probably the best one for the job but it is not necessarily a truer or more real description of the United Kingdom than a map showing annual rainfall.

The point I am trying to make is that the map is not the terrain. The Western biological map of the human body is only one potentially useful medical map. It is no more true than the traditional Chinese medical map and the facts of one map cannot be reduced to the criteria or standards of another unless they share the same logic right from the beginning. As long as the Western medical map is capable of solving a person's disease in a cost-effective, time-efficient manner without side-effects or iatrogenesis (disease or illness caused by treatment), then it is a useful map. Chinese medicine needs to be judged in the same way. The Chinese medical map of health and disease is just as 'real' and every bit as useful as the Western biological map as long as in using it practitioners and patients are able to solve health problems in a safe and effective way.

The following chapter is an introduction to the fundamental concepts of Chinese medicine. Once you have a basic understanding of some of these fundamental concepts you will be able to appreciate how Chinese medicine may help in the treatment of depression.

AN OVERVIEW OF THE CHINESE MEDICAL MAP

In this chapter we will present an overview of Chinese medicine. In particular, we will discuss yin and yang, qi and blood, essence and spirit, the viscera and bowels and the channels and network vessels. In the following chapter, we will also look at the concept of qi stagnation and the relationship between both the menstrual cycle and ageing and qi stagnation. Once we understand these concepts, we can then go on to see how Chinese medicine views depression and how a practitioner of Chinese medicine is able to diagnose and treat a person suffering from depression. Should you find any of the language or terms used to describe Chinese medicine difficult to understand, there is a glossary on pages 161–6 to which you can refer.

YIN AND YANG

To understand Chinese medicine, one must first understand the concepts of yin and yang, since these are the most basic in this system. Yin and yang are the cornerstones for understanding, diagnosing and treating the body and mind in Chinese medicine. In a sense, all the other theories and concepts of Chinese medicine are simply an elaboration of yin and yang. Most people have probably already heard of yin and yang but may not have a clear idea of what these terms mean.

The concepts of yin and yang can be used to describe everything that exists in the universe, including all the parts and functions of the body. Originally, yin referred to the shady side of a hill and yang to the sunny side of the hill. Since sunshine and shade are two interdependent sides of a single reality, these two aspects of the hill are seen as part of a single whole. Other examples of yin and yang are that night exists only in relation to day and cold exists only in relation to heat. According to Chinese thought, every single thing that exists in the universe has these two aspects, a yin and a yang. Thus everything has a front and a back, a top and a bottom, a left and a right and a beginning and an end. However, something is yin or yang only in relation to its paired complement. Nothing is of itself yin or yang.

It is the concepts of yin and yang that make Chinese medicine a holistic medicine. This is because, based on this unitary and complementary vision of reality, no body part or body function is viewed as separate or isolated from the whole person. The table below shows a partial list of yin and yang pairs as they apply to the body. It is vital to remember that each item listed is either yin or yang only in relation to its complementary partner. Nothing is absolutely or within itself either yin or yang. As we can see from the list, it is possible to describe every aspect of the body in terms of yin and yang.

Yin	Yang
Form	Function
Organs	Bowels
Blood	Qi
Inside	Outside
Front of body	Back of body
Right side	Left side
Lower body	Upper body
Cool, cold	Warm, hot
Stillness	Activity, movement

QI AND BLOOD

Qi (pronounced chee) and blood make up the most important complementary pair of yin and yang within the human body. It is said that in the world yin and yang are water and fire, but in the human body, yin and yang are blood and qi. Qi is yang in relation to blood, which is yin.

Qi

Qi is often translated as energy and certainly energy is a manifestation of qi. Chinese language scholars would say, however, that qi is larger than any single type of energy described by modern Western science. Paul Unschuld, in my opinion one of the greatest living sinologists, translates the word qi as influences. This conveys the sense that qi is what is responsible for change and movement. So with regard to Chinese medicine, qi is that which motivates all movement and transformation or change.

In Chinese medicine, qi is defined as having five specific functions:

1. Defence

It is qi that is responsible for protecting the exterior of the body from invasion by external pathogens. This form of qi, which is called defensive qi, flows through the exterior or outer portion of the body.

2. Transformation

Qi transforms substances so that they can be utilised by the body. An example of this function is the transformation of the food we eat into nutrients to nourish the body, which then produces more qi and blood.

3. Warming

Qi, being relatively yang, is inherently warm, and one of the main functions of the qi is to warm the entire body, both inside and out. If this warming function of the qi is weak, then the lack of warmth and resulting cold may cause the flow of qi and blood to become congealed in a similar way to the effect of cold on water – freezing.

4. Restraint

It is the qi that holds all the organs and substances of the body in their proper place. All the organs, blood and fluids need qi to keep them from falling or leaking out of their specific pathways. If this function of the qi is weak, then problems like uterine prolapse, a tendency to bruise easily or urinary incontinence may occur.

5. Transportation

Qi provides the motivating force for all transportation and movement in the body. Every aspect of the body that moves is moved by the qi. The qi moves the blood and body fluids throughout the body. It moves food through the stomach and blood through the vessels.

Blood

In Chinese medicine, as in modern Western medicine, blood refers to the red fluid that flows through our vessels but it also has different meanings and implications. Most basically, blood is the substance that nourishes and moistens all the body tissues. Without blood, body tissues cannot function properly. Additionally, when there is insufficient blood or it is scanty, body tissues become dry and wither.

Qi and blood are closely interrelated. In Chinese medicine it is said, 'Qi is the commander of the blood and blood is the mother of qi'. This means that it is qi that moves the blood but it is the blood that provides the nourishment and physical foundation for the creation and existence of the qi.

In Chinese medicine, blood provides the following functions for the body:

1. Nourishment

Blood nourishes the body. Along with qi, the blood goes to every part of the body. If the blood is deficient, function decreases and tissues atrophy or shrink.

2. Moistening

Blood moistens the body tissues. This includes the skin, eyes and ligaments and tendons or what are simply called the sinews of the body in Chinese medicine. Blood deficiency can cause drying out and consequent stiffening of various body tissues throughout the body.

3. Material foundation for the spirit or mind

In Chinese medicine, the body and mind are considered as one. The blood (yin) supplies the material support and nourishment for the mind (yang) allowing it to become 'bright' (i.e. conscious and clever) and stay rooted in the body. If blood is insufficient, the mind can 'float', causing problems like insomnia, agitation and unrest.

ESSENCE

Along with qi and blood, essence is one of the three most important constituents of the body. Essence is the most fundamental, essential material the body uses for its growth, maturation and reproduction. There are two forms of this essence: there is the essence we inherit from our parents and there is the essence we produce from the food and drink that we consume and the air we breathe.

The essence that comes from our parents is what determines our basic constitution, strength and vitality. We each have a finite, limited amount of this inherited essence. It is important to protect and conserve this essence because all bodily functions depend upon it, and when it is gone we die. The depletion of essence has serious implications for our overall health and well-being. Fortunately, the essence derived from food and drink helps to bolster and support this inherited essence. So, if we eat well and do not consume more qi and blood than we create each day, then when we sleep at night this surplus qi and, more especially, blood are transformed into essence.

SPIRIT

Spirit in Chinese medicine refers to mental and emotional faculties. Fundamentally, spirit refers to consciousness. From a modern Chinese medical perspective, this term does not have any religious or 'spiritual' connotations. Spirit in a Chinese medical sense is simply considered to be an accumulation of qi and blood in the heart. When sufficient qi and blood have accumulated in the heart, then this gives rise to consciousness, which in Chinese medicine is called the spirit. Sometimes different terms are used to describe specific aspects of the spirit. Due to a close interrelationship between the essence, the qi and the spirit, sometimes consciousness is called the 'essence spirit'. If we are talking about the emotions in particular, then the compound term 'spirit will' (will meaning desire) is commonly used. At other times, since the spirit is associated with mental clarity, the compound term 'spirit brightness' or 'spirit brilliance' is used.

In order for spirit to be present at all, there must be sufficient qi. For the spirit to be calm and healthy, there must be sufficient blood as it nourishes the spirit and keeps it rooted or under control. The spirit made from qi is inherently yang in nature and it tends to stir or become restless if yin blood does not nourish and 'mother' it. Normal mental clarity is referred to as 'having spirit', while emotional upset may lead to a state of agitation and be referred to as 'spirit not quiet' or 'restless spirit'.

On the one hand, the spirit is made up from the qi and blood that are produced by the viscera and bowels, which we will talk about next. On the other, the qi, and consequently the spirit, are affected by external stimuli. There is no dichotomy or division in Chinese medicine between the psychological and biological. The mind and consciousness arise as a function of the viscera and bowels, which in turn are affected by the experiences of the mind and emotions. Every thought we formulate or emotion we feel is considered to be simply the experience of the movement of qi. If we change the way the qi moves, we can change our mental–emotional experience and, conversely, if we change our mind and emotions this will affect the movement of qi. The qi and the spirit or mind are not two different things but aspects of a single reality or whole.

THE VISCERA AND BOWELS

In Chinese medicine, the internal organs (called viscera so as not to become confused with the Western biological entities of the same name) have a much wider area of function and influence than in Western medicine. Each viscus has distinct responsibilities for maintaining the physical and psychological health of the individual. From a Chinese medical perspective, it is more useful to view each viscus as a sphere of influence or a network that spreads throughout the body, rather than as the distinct and separate physical organ that is described in Western science. It is for this reason that the renowned German sinologist Manfred Porkert refers to the viscera as orbs rather than as organs. In Chinese medicine, the relationship and connections between the various viscera and other parts of the body are facilitated by the channel and network vessel system that we will discuss below.

According to Chinese medicine, there are five main viscera that are relatively yin and six main bowels that are relatively yang. The five yin viscera are the heart, lungs, liver, spleen and kidneys. The six yang bowels are the stomach, small intestine, large intestine, gall bladder, urinary bladder and a system that Chinese medicine refers to as the triple burner. The functions of the entire body are categorised or described under these eleven organs or spheres of influence. Chinese medicine as a system does not have a pancreas, a pituitary gland or ovaries, as their functions and others are described by the sphere of influence of the five viscera and six bowels. The actual functions of the viscera and bowels are more important and wider-reaching than their physical structure. For example, someone who had had their gall bladder removed would still have the functional aspects of the gall bladder from the point of view of Chinese medicine available to them.

Within this system, the five viscera are the most important. These are the organs that in Chinese medicine are responsible for the creation and transformation of qi and blood and the storage of essence. The kidneys, for example, are responsible for the excretion of urine, but in addition they have many other areas of responsibility or spheres of influence, such as hearing, bone strength, sex, reproduction, maturation and growth, the lower and upper back, the lower legs in general and the knees in particular.

Visceral correspondences

The Chinese viscera may have the same name and even some functions in common with the organs of modern Western medicine, but they are quite different from them.

Each of the five Chinese medical viscera also has a corresponding tissue, sense and emotion related to it. These are outlined in the table below.

Organ	Tissue	Sense	Spirit	Emotion
Lungs	Skin/body hair	Smell	Corporeal soul	Grief/sadness
Spleen	Flesh	Taste	Thought	Thinking/worry
Kidneys	Bones/head hair	Hearing	Will	Fear
Liver	Sinews	Sight	Ethereal soul	Anger
Heart	Blood vessels	Speech	Spirit	Joy/fright

Each Chinese medical viscus or bowel possesses both a yin and a yang aspect. The yin aspect of a viscus or bowel refers to its substantial nature or tangible form. Furthermore, an organ's yin is responsible for the nurturing, cooling and moistening of that viscus or bowel. The yang aspect of the viscus or bowel represents its functional activities or what it does. An organ's yang aspect is also warming. These two aspects, yin and yang, form and function, cooling and heating, create good health when balanced. If either yin or yang becomes too strong or too weak, the resulting imbalance may lead to disease.

All five viscera have potential associations with the causes and mechanisms of depression, whilst only two of the six bowels may be involved, namely the gall bladder and stomach. We will now look further at the workings of these five viscera and two bowels and how they relate to the diagnosis and treatment of depression in Chinese medicine.

The kidneys

In Chinese medicine, the kidneys are considered to be the foundation of our life. Since the developing foetus is shaped like a kidney and because the kidneys are the main viscus for the storage of our inherited essence, the kidneys are referred to as the prenatal root. Keeping the kidney qi strong and kidney yin and yang in relative balance is considered essential to good health and longevity. The Chinese medical aspects relating to the kidneys that are most relevant to the mechanisms of depression are:

1. Human reproduction, development and maturation

These are the same functions we referred to when describing the essence. This is because the essence is said to be stored in the kidneys. Health problems related to reproduction, development and maturation are commonly problems of the kidney essence. Excessive sexual activity, drug use or simple prolonged over-exhaustion can all damage and consume kidney essence. Kidney essence is also consumed by the simple process of ageing.

2. Foundation of water metabolism

The kidneys work in co-ordination with the lungs and spleen to ensure that water is spread properly throughout the body and that excess water is excreted as urine. Problems such as oedema, excessive dryness or excessive day- or night-time urination can indicate a weakness of kidney function.

3. Storing the will

Will in this sense refers to desire. If kidney qi is insufficient, this aspect of our human nature can be weakened. Pushing ourselves to physical extremes, such as long-distance running or cycling, can eventually exhaust our kidneys.

4. Fear

Fear can result when the kidney qi is insufficient. On the other hand, constant or excessive fear can damage the kidneys and make them weak.

The liver

In Chinese medicine, the liver is associated with emotional state, with digestion and with menstruation in women. Specifically, its functions include:

1. Coursing and discharge

Coursing and discharge refer to the uninhibited spreading of qi to every part of the body. If the liver is not able to maintain the free and smooth flow of qi throughout the body, multiple physical and emotional symptoms can develop. This function of the liver is most easily damaged by emotional causes and, in particular, by anger and frustration. For example, if the liver is stressed due to pent-up anger, the flow of liver qi can become depressed or stagnate.

Liver qi stagnation can cause a wide range of health

problems, including PMS, chronic digestive disturbance, depression and insomnia. Therefore, it is essential to keep our liver qi flowing freely.

2. Storing the blood

This means that the liver regulates the amount of blood in circulation. In particular, when the body is at rest, the blood in the extremities returns to the liver. As an extension of this, it is said in Chinese medicine that the liver is yin in form but yang in function. The liver requires sufficient blood to keep it and its associated tissues moist and supple, cool and relaxed.

3. Anger

Anger is the emotion that typically arises when the liver is diseased and especially when its qi does not flow freely. Conversely, anger damages the liver. The emotions related to the stagnation of qi in the liver are frustration, anger and rage.

The heart

Although the heart is the emperor of the body–mind according to Chinese medicine, it does not play as large a role in the creation and treatment of disease as one might think. Rather than the emperor initiating the cause of disease, enduring disease usually eventually affects the heart. Especially in terms of depression, disturbances of the heart tend to be secondary rather than primary. By this I mean that some other viscus or bowel becomes diseased first and then the heart feels the negative effect. The Chinese medical concept of the heart has the following specific functions that relate to depression:

1. Governing the blood

This means that it is the heart qi that 'stirs' or moves the blood within its vessels. This is roughly analogous to the heart pumping the blood in Western medicine. The pulsation of the blood through the arteries due to the contraction of the heart is referred to as the 'stirring of the pulse'. In fact, the Chinese word for pulse and vessel is the same. So this could also be translated as the 'stirring of the vessels'.

2. Storing the spirit

The spirit refers to the mind in Chinese medicine. This statement underscores the fact that mental function, clarity and equilibrium are all associated with the heart. If the heart does not receive enough qi or blood or if the heart is disturbed by something, the spirit may become restless and this may produce symptoms of mental and emotional unrest, heart palpitations, insomnia and profuse dreams.

3. Governing the vessels

This concept is very close to point 1 above. The vessels refer to the blood vessels and also to the pulse.

4. Governing speech

If heart function becomes abnormal, this may be reflected in various speech problems such as stuttering or raving and delirious speech, muttering to oneself and speaking incoherently.

5. Portal of the tongue

The heart has a special relationship with the tongue, especially its tip. Heart problems may manifest as sores on the tip of the tongue.

6. Joy

The emotion of joy helps to ease the flow of qi (and therefore blood). It helps us to relax and we feel more harmonious. The emotion of joy is very healing, as is laughter. Joy and laughter are associated with the heart. If there is too much joy, such as when someone becomes over-excited, this can be damaging to the heart. It is interesting to look at manic depression in terms of these polar opposites: the person is flat, emotionless and depressed on the one hand, but manic and wildly excited on the other. It is also interesting that many famous comedians have died of heart attacks or suffered from depression – Peter Sellers, Tommy Cooper and Tony Hancock, for example.

The spleen

In Chinese medicine, the spleen plays a pivotal role in the creation of qi and blood and also in the circulation and transformation of body fluids. The role of the spleen in Chinese medicine is very wide-reaching and more important than in Western medicine. This is an excellent illustration of how these two systems of medicine differ in their views of the internal organs and their functions. According to Chinese medicine, the main functions of the spleen that relate to depression are:

1. Movement and transformation

This refers to the movement and transformation of foods and liquids through the digestive system. In this case, movement and transformation may be considered to be digestion. Movement and transformation may also refer to the movement and transformation of body fluids through the body. It is the spleen qi that is largely responsible for controlling liquid metabolism in the body.

2. Restraining the blood

As mentioned before, one of the five functions of the qi is to restrain the fluids of the body, including the blood, within their proper channels and reservoirs. If the spleen qi is healthy and abundant, then the blood is properly held within its vessels. Conversely, if the spleen qi becomes weak and insufficient, then the blood may flow outside its channels and vessels, resulting in various types of pathological bleeding, including those associated with the menstrual cycle.

3. Storing the constructive

The constructive is one of the types of qi in the body. Specifically, it is the qi responsible for nourishing and constructing the body and its tissues. This constructive qi is closely associated with the process of digestion and the creation of qi and blood from food and liquids. If the spleen fails to store, or runs out of, constructive qi, then the person first becomes hungry and eventually fatigued.

4. Thought

In the West, we do not usually consider the process of thought as an emotion per se. However, in Chinese medicine it is classified as an emotion along with anger, joy, fear, grief and melancholy. In particular, thinking, or perhaps I should say over-thinking or obsessive thinking, causes the spleen qi to 'bind'. The result may be that the spleen qi does not flow harmoniously and can typically manifest in such symptoms as loss of appetite, abdominal bloating after meals and indigestion.

5. Engenderment and transformation

Engenderment and transformation refer to the creation or production of the qi and blood out of the food and drink we take in each day. If the spleen receives adequate food and drink and then properly transforms that food and drink, it engenders, or creates, the qi and blood. Whilst the kidneys and lungs also participate in the creation of the qi, and the kidneys and heart participate in the creation of the blood, the spleen is the pivotal viscus in both processes. Spleen qi weakness and insufficiency is one of the main causes of qi and blood deficiency and weakness.

The lungs

The lungs are perhaps not as important in relation to depression as the other Chinese viscera. Like the heart, the lungs often bear the brunt of disease processes initiated in other viscera and bowels. As in Western medicine, the lungs are often subject to external invading pathogens resulting in respiratory tract diseases. From a Chinese medical perspective, the lungs' sphere of influence also includes the skin and fluid metabolism. The main functions of the lungs according to Chinese medicine are as follows:

1. Governing the qi

Specifically, the lungs govern the downward spread and circulation of the qi. It is the lung qi that moves all the rest of the qi in the body out to the edges and from the top of the body downwards. The lung qi is like a sprinkler spraying out qi. This downward qi ensures body fluids are moved throughout the body, down to the kidneys and bladder and, eventually, out of the body.

2. Governing the defensive exterior

We said above that the qi defends the body against invasion from external pathogens. In Chinese medicine, the outermost layer of the body is the area where the defensive qi circulates and the place where this defence takes place first. It is the lungs that govern this defensive qi. If the lungs function normally and there is sufficient defensive qi, then the body is protected from invasion by external pathogens. If the lungs are weak and the defensive qi is insufficient, then external pathogens may easily invade the exterior of the body, causing complaints such as colds, flu and allergies.

The gall bladder

In Chinese medicine the main functions of the gall bladder in terms of depression are:

1. Governing decision

In Chinese medicine, the liver is likened to a general who plans strategy for the body, while the gall bladder is likened to a judge. According to this point of view, if a person lacks gall bladder qi, they will have trouble making decisions. As well as being indecisive they may also be timid and hesitant. While courage in the West is most often associated with the heart (from *coeur*, the French for heart, we get courage), bravery in the East is most often associated with the gall bladder. Actually, this is also an old Western idea too. When someone is very forward and brazen, we say that they have gall. Conversely, if someone is excessively timid, this may be due to gall bladder qi vacuity or insufficiency. In Chinese medicine, this is called 'gall bladder timidity'. An inability to make decisions is common in people suffering with depression, as well as a lack of confidence and feelings of insecurity.

2. The liver and gall bladder are a yin–yang pair

This statement underscores the particularly close relationship between the liver and gall bladder.

3. The eleven viscera depend on the gall bladder

4. If there is qi because of a robust gall bladder, evils are not able to enter

These last two statements about the gall bladder are very similar to statements in Chinese medicine about the heart, that say that the heart is the sovereign of the body and that if spirit abides (in the heart), then evils cannot enter. Both these statements elevate the gall bladder to a place of importance in the body it does not hold in Western medicine and, in a way, link the gall bladder to the heart and its spirit.

The stomach

There are a number of important functions that relate to the stomach in Chinese medicine due to the stomach's pivotal role in digestion and, therefore, in the creation of qi and blood. Here we will discuss only those functions that will be useful in our discussion of the disease causes and disease mechanisms of depression in Chinese medicine.

1. The stomach governs intake

This means that the stomach is the first to receive foods and drinks ingested into the body.

2. The stomach governs the bearing down of the turbid

The process of digestion in Chinese medicine is likened to the process of fermentation and then distillation. The stomach is the fermentation vat wherein foods and liquids rot and ripen. This allows for the separation of clear and turbid parts of the digested food. The spleen sends the clear parts upwards to the lungs and heart to become the qi and blood respectively. The stomach's job is to send the turbid part down to be excreted as waste from the large intestine and bladder.

3. Stomach heat may exploit the heart

If abnormal or pathological heat collects in the stomach it may affect the heart. As heat is yang and has an innate tendency to move upwards and outwards and as the heart is located above the stomach in Chinese medicine, heat in the stomach may exploit or harass the heart situated above it.

4. The stomach is the origin of defensive qi

We have seen earlier that the defensive qi is the qi that defends the exterior of the body from invasion by external pathogens. The defensive qi has another job, which is to warm the internal organs. According to some points of view, the stomach is the origin of the defensive qi. This is because it is in the stomach that the clear and turbid parts of the digested food are separated, and the defensive qi is made out of a further refinement of the turbid part of this.

Triple burner

We mentioned that there are five viscera and six bowels. The sixth bowel is called the triple burner. It is said in Chinese medicine, 'The triple burner has a function but no form.' The name triple burner refers to the three main areas of the torso.

The upper burner is the chest. The middle burner is the space from the bottom of the ribcage to the level of the navel. The lower burner is the lower abdomen below the navel. These three spaces are called burners because all of the functions and transformations of the viscera and bowels which they contain are 'warm' transformations, similar to food cooking in a pot on a stove or to an alchemical transformation in a furnace. In fact, the triple burner is simply a generalised concept of how the other viscera and bowels function together as an organic unit in terms of the digestion of foods and liquids and the circulation and transformation of body fluids.

As we will see below there are channels or meridians connected with each viscus and each bowel. There is a channel, however, that is very important in the treatment of depression, that does not correspond to any viscera or bowel. This channel, the *hand jue yin* channel, known in English as the pericardium or heart protector, functions both as an extension of the heart in relation to the spirit and as a regulator of the flow of qi mediated by the liver in the upper and middle burners.

THE CHANNELS AND NETWORK VESSELS

Each viscus and bowel has a corresponding channel or meridian with which it is connected. In Chinese medicine, the inside of the body is made up of the viscera and bowels. The outside of the body is composed of the sinews, bones, muscles, flesh, skin and hair. It is the channels and network vessels (i.e. smaller connecting vessels) that connect the inside and the outside of the body. It is through these channels and network vessels that the viscera and bowels connect with their corresponding body tissues.

The channel and network vessel system is a unique feature of Chinese medicine. These channels and vessels are different from the circulatory, nervous or lymphatic systems. The earliest reference to these channels and vessels is in *Nei*

Jing (The Inner Classic), a text written around the second or third century BC.

The channels and vessels perform two basic functions. They are the pathways by which the qi and blood circulate through the body and between the organs and tissues. Additionally, as mentioned above, the channels connect the viscera and bowels with the exterior part of the body. This channel and vessel system functions in the body much like an information or communication network. The channels allow the various parts of our bodies to co-operate and interact to maintain our lives.

This channel and network vessel system is quite complex. There are 12 primary channels, six yin and six yang, each with a specific pathway through the external body and connected with an internal organ (see diagram overleaf). There are also extraordinary vessels, sinew channels, channel divergences, main network vessels and ultimately countless finer and finer network vessels permeating the entire body. All of these form a closed loop or circuit similar to but distinct from the Western circulatory system.

Acupuncture points are places located on the major channels where there is a special concentration of qi and blood. As there is relatively more qi and blood accumulated at these points, the sites act as switches, which can potentially influence the flow of qi and blood in the relative channel. By stimulating these points in any of a number of different ways, one can speed up or slow down, increase or reduce, warm or cool the qi and blood flowing in the channels and vessels. The main methods used to stimulate these points and adjust the flow of qi and blood in the channels and vessels are acupuncture (see page 88) and moxibustion (see page 119). Other commonly used ways of stimulating these points and thus adjusting the qi and blood flowing through the channels and vessels are massage, cupping, the application of magnets and the application of various herbal medicinals. If the channels and vessels are the pathways over which the qi and

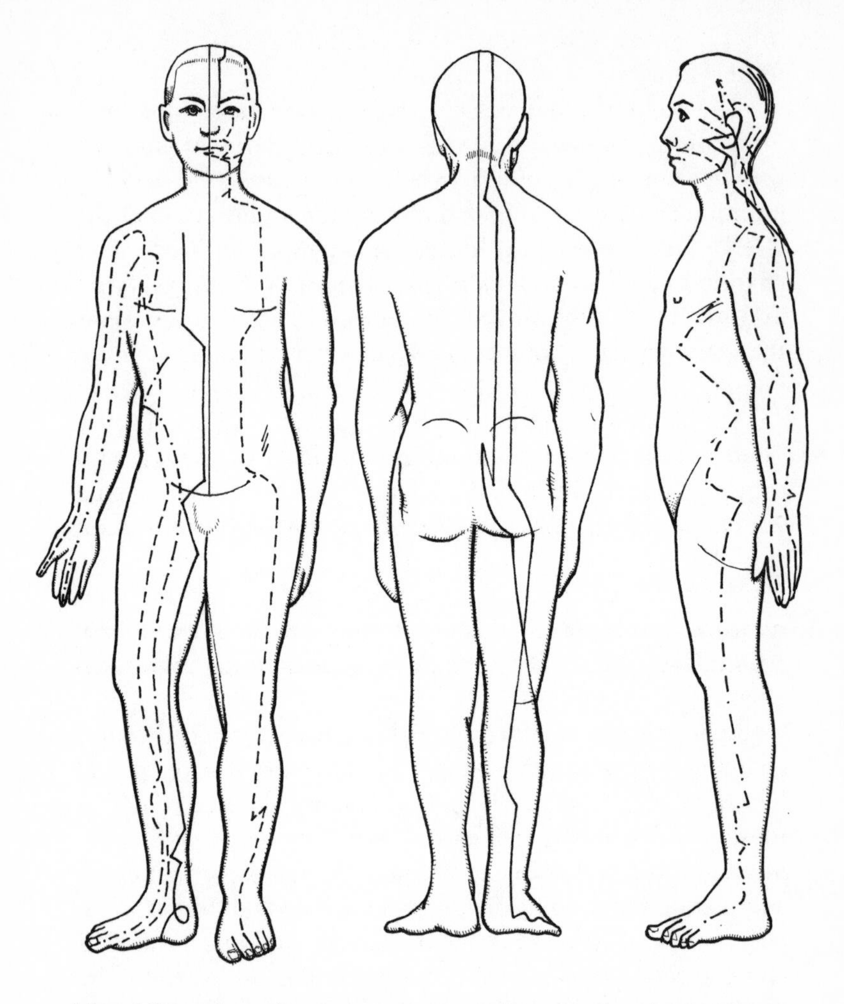

blood flow, then the acupuncture points are the places where this flow can be adjusted.

THE CONCEPT OF QI STAGNATION AND ITS RELATIONSHIP TO THE LIVER

As we will soon see, the concept of qi stagnation, which we mentioned earlier, is essential to the understanding of the Chinese mechanisms of depression. This chapter will focus on a discussion of the causes and ramifications of qi stagnation. In particular, we will also look at qi stagnation from the point of view of the female menstrual cycle and see how ageing affects qi stagnation in both men and women.

As we saw above, the liver spreads the qi and maintains the smooth and unobstructed flow of qi. Since the qi moves the blood, this smooth and uninhibited flow of qi ensures the free and easy flow of blood. It is said in Chinese medicine that 'The liver is the temperamental viscus' and that 'The liver likes to spread freely'. This means that the liver is typically the first viscus or organ negatively affected by mental–emotional stress and frustrations. If the liver is negatively affected by frustration, suppressed emotion or stress, its functions will be affected. In this situation, the qi does not spread freely throughout the body, but rather becomes stagnant. Technically, in Chinese medicine this is referred to as liver depression qi stagnation and its main cause is emotional stress and frustration.

Throughout this book the word depression is used in two different but related ways. When occurring alone, the word depression primarily means the Western disease of depression. When combined with the word liver, as in liver depression qi stagnation, it refers to a particular Chinese disease mechanism and pattern of disharmony. Although it is our thesis that the overwhelming majority of sufferers of the disease depression manifest, at least in part, the Chinese pattern of liver depression qi stagnation, there is no direct correlation between these two concepts. As we will see below, liver depression is only one contributing factor in most people's depression, even if it is a pivotal one.

ACCUMULATION AND COUNTERFLOW

If the liver becomes depressed and the qi consequently becomes stagnant, the qi will tend to back up and accumulate, as it has to go somewhere. The result is that one of the first symptoms of qi stagnation is fullness and distension in the areas traversed by the channels and vessels connected to the liver. The liver channel traverses or connects with the insides of the legs and thighs, the pelvic region, the upper abdomen, the chest, the throat, gums, eyes and top of the head. The liver channel is connected to the *hand jue yin* pericardium channel, a sort of extension of the liver channel in the upper part of the body. This channel traverses the insides of the arms but especially the upper abdomen and the chest. The liver channel also connects with the gall bladder channel. The gall bladder channel is the yang channel paired to the yin liver channel. The course of the gall bladder channel runs up the outsides of the legs, through the pelvis, up the sides of the flanks, the sides of the neck and the sides of the head. Since qi is yang, stagnant and therefore accumulated qi, which originates in a yin viscus and channel, often moves into its paired yang channel. So the symptoms of liver depression qi stagnation often manifest as fullness, distension and lack of free flow on the gall bladder channel. Additionally, as the qi is yang, it has an innate tendency to move in the yang direction – upwards. If the qi becomes stagnant and accumulates, it will eventually flow upwards, and it may also flow horizontally as well.

DEPRESSIVE HEAT

There is yet another consequence of the qi being yang when it becomes depressed and stagnant. What happens to air that is pumped into a tyre as the pressure in that tyre begins to mount? It becomes hot. If enough qi becomes trapped and depressed, it will eventually transform into heat. This heat is technically called depressive heat in Chinese medicine. It is the result of extreme or long-term stagnation of the liver qi. In summary, there are three main groups of symptoms associated with liver depression qi stagnation due to emotional stress and frustration: fullness and distension, counterflow (i.e. the venting of excessive liver qi to an area of the body it should not be in) and depressive or transformative heat. As heat typically moves upwards due to its inherently yang nature, this depressive heat may negatively affect the function of the organs and tissues located above the liver. These include the stomach, heart and lungs in terms of viscera and bowels, and the head, mouth, nose, ears and eyes in terms of body parts. Since the spirit is said to reside in the heart, upwardly counterflowing depressive heat may disturb the heart spirit, causing it to become 'restless'.

QI STAGNATION AND THE BLOOD AND BODY FLUIDS

If the qi is not circulating freely it is unable to move and transform the blood and body fluids, which then also begin to stagnate. Long-term qi stagnation may result in blood stasis and the accumulation of dampness. If dampness lingers and is not transformed, it may congeal into phlegm. This phlegm may then lodge in the viscera or bowels, the channels or network vessels or in the body's various orifices, further obstructing the flow of qi and, therefore, the function of those viscera, channels or orifices. Similarly, blood stasis, dampness accumulation or phlegm obstruction occurring for any reason may cause or aggravate qi stagnation. Once these pathological yin substances exist in the body, they hinder and impede the free and easy flow of yang qi. Thus, qi stagnation may give rise to blood stasis, dampness or phlegm, while blood stasis, dampness and phlegm may cause or aggravate qi stagnation.

THE MENSTRUAL CYCLE IN CHINESE MEDICINE

Statistically, more women suffer from depression than men.[2] Interestingly, there are some Chinese theories that explain this situation. In Chinese medicine it is said that men and women are basically the same. Women, however, have a uterus; they menstruate, and can conceive, give birth and lactate. The fact that more women are diagnosed with depression is considered to be due to the mechanics of their menstrual cycle *vis-à-vis* liver depression qi stagnation.

The menses themselves are a discharge of blood. For this discharge to take place, two things have to occur. Firstly, a superabundance of blood must accumulate in the uterus for it eventually to spill over as menstruation. Secondly, the qi and blood must be freely and uninhibitedly flowing in order to allow this brimming over. This means that in order to understand menstruation, an understanding of how blood is created and what might affect the free and uninhibited flow of qi and blood is needed.

The creation of blood

There are three viscera that participate in the creation of the blood. These are the kidneys, spleen and heart. The heart is the place where the blood is 'turned red' or finally created. However, first the spleen must send up the finest essence of food and liquids extracted in the process of digestion. If the spleen does not send up this finest essence of food and liquids

---

[2] *The Merck Manual of Diagnosis and Therapy*, ed. Robert Berkow, Merck, Sharp and Dohme Research Laboratories, Rahway, New Jersey, 1987.

there will be insufficient supplies for the heart to transform these into blood. Additionally, the kidneys must send up some essence to participate in the creation of blood.

So if the kidneys lack sufficient essence, if the spleen fails to digest the finest essence of food and liquids and send this upwards or if the heart, for any reason, cannot fulfil its function of 'turning the blood red', then there may be insufficient creation of blood. In addition, it is the heart's job to spread the blood to the rest of the body and eventually move it down to the uterus. It is said in Chinese medicine that first the blood goes to nourish and moisten the viscera and bowels and then it goes into the channels and vessels. From there it nourishes and moistens the rest of the tissues of the body and what collects in the uterus is what is left over after the blood has performed all these other jobs. When enough blood collects in the uterus to fill it, it overflows as the menses. Typically, a young to middle-aged, healthy woman will produce such a superabundance accumulating in the uterus once every 28–30 days.

The control of the blood

Although normal menstruation cannot occur if there is insufficient blood accumulated in the uterus, it can occur either too early or too late if the flow of blood is not controlled properly. Just as there are three viscera that create and transform the blood, there are three viscera that 'govern' or 'control' the blood. These are the heart, liver and spleen. It is said that the heart qi governs the blood. As explained above, this means that it is the heart qi that 'stirs' or pushes the blood. If the heart qi does not move the blood, the blood cannot move on its own. Thus it is said, 'If the qi moves, the blood moves. If the qi stops, the blood stops.'

In actual fact, the heart gets its qi primarily from the spleen. So a sufficiency of spleen qi is necessary for there to be enough heart qi to move the blood. In addition, the spleen qi restrains and contains the blood within its channels and vessels. If the spleen qi is too weak, it may allow the blood to seep out prematurely or it may not cut off menstruation when it should. Finally, the liver stores the blood. It is the liver's job to regulate the amount of blood in circulation. It is the liver qi that performs this function. If the liver qi spreads freely, then the blood moves. If the liver qi becomes depressed and stagnant, then the blood will also eventually become depressed and static.

One may find it hard at first to distinguish between the spleen's role and the liver's role in maintaining the free and uninhibited flow of blood. It is ultimately the spleen qi (via the heart) that provides the motivating force behind the propulsion of the blood. It is the liver that allows the blood to flow freely through its channels and vessels. If, for instance, you have petrol in your car and the car is in good working order, the power is available to move the car. However, if you are stopped at a red light, you do not have the permission to move the car even though the power is there. In terms of the heart, spleen and liver, the flow of blood is the same. The heart and spleen provide the motivating power, but it is the liver qi that determines whether that blood flows freely or not.

If for any reason one of these three viscera does not function correctly in terms of the flow of blood, this may impede the free and timely flow of the menstruate. Conversely, the menstrual cycle places certain burdens on and affects these viscera in ways not experienced by men. The functions of the liver, heart, spleen and kidneys may all be negatively impacted by the menstrual cycle and, as we shall see below, these are the main viscera involved in depression.

The four phases of the menstrual cycle

Chinese medicine divides the menstrual cycle into four periods of roughly seven days. Phase one begins the day the menses end. Counting the days of the menstrual cycle from the first day of the onset of menstruation, this means that phase one typically begins on day four, five, six or seven. The uterus has discharged its accumulated blood and this leaves the body relatively empty or vacuous of blood. Since the blood is created, at least in part, out of kidney essence, and because, compared to yang qi, essence is a type of yin substance, during phase one the body busies itself with making more yin blood to replenish that which was discharged. Therefore, we say that phase one corresponds to yin and the emphasis in the body is on replenishing yin blood.

If the body is having a hard time replacing this blood due to kidney yin vacuity, the heart spirit may not receive enough blood to nourish it and thus it may become more restless than usual during this phase. Since yin controls yang, yang heat may flare upward to harass the spirit in the heart and the spirit may also become restless for this reason.

Phase two corresponds to the days surrounding ovulation. Until now, the body has been replenishing its yin. However, for ovulation to occur, yin must transform into yang. This transformation of yin into yang corresponds to the rise in basal body temperature which occurs after ovulation.[3] If there is insufficient yin, it cannot transform into yang. Conversely, if there is insufficient yang, it cannot transform yin. In addition, if either the qi or blood is not flowing freely, this transformation may also be impeded. Generally, phase two relates to days 10–16 in the monthly cycle and it corresponds to yang in the same way that phase one corresponds to yin.

If yin has grown successfully during phase one, the growth of yang may begin to progress during phase two. Since yang is associated with heat, this means that yang heat may flare upwards, disturbing the heart spirit and causing restlessness and agitation. In this case, heat added to liver depression may cause otherwise simple qi stagnation to turn into depressive

---

[3] Basal body temperature refers to resting temperature when taken the first thing upon waking in the morning before getting up, dressing, eating, or doing anything else. It is analogous to resting pulse or basal metabolic rate. Plotting basal body temperature on a graph is one way of determining if and when a woman is ovulating.

heat or even fire. What was irritability may thus become irascibility, while feelings of fullness, distension and oppression may all become aggravated by a vexatious feeling of heat and agitation or restlessness.

Phase three corresponds to the premenstruum and to the qi. For the woman's body to function as it should, yang qi must stay strong enough long enough and the qi must flow freely and in the right direction. Many of the signs and symptoms of premenstrual syndrome (PMS), including premenstrual depression or a worsening of chronic depression during this time every month, have to do with the yang qi not being strong enough or the qi (and therefore the blood) not flowing freely.

The yang qi is produced by the spleen and kidneys. If for any reason, such as improper diet, excessive work, insufficient exercise, enduring disease, too much thinking and anxiety (spleen), too much fear (kidneys) or simply ageing, the spleen and/or kidneys become weak, symptoms such as fatigue, lack of will, listlessness and somnolence may occur or worsen during the premenstruum when extra strains are placed on the functions of these two viscera.

Additionally, because the liver's function of coursing and discharge is dependent on nourishment of the liver by the blood, if a woman has too little blood, when the blood she does have accumulates in the uterus prior to menstruation, this may leave the rest of her body 'high and dry'. That means liver function may be compromised, thus causing or worsening liver depression qi stagnation. It also means that the heart spirit may not receive its proper nourishment from the blood, which causes it to become unquiet or restless. Therefore, there are a number of reasons why a woman might become more depressed and/or agitated during phase three of her menstrual cycle. Phase three is usually counted from day 17 to the day before menstruation. However, in real life, phase three begins whenever a woman begins to feel the onset of cyclically recurring PMS.

Phase four is the menstruation itself. Since the onset of menstruation is counted as day one in the cycle, phase four may last anywhere from one or two days to six or seven, depending on the individual woman's constitution and age. Since menstruation is a downward discharge of blood according to Chinese medicine, phase four corresponds to the blood. Typically, this discharge of blood and the qi that follows along with it is experienced as a reduction in any signs and symptoms associated with liver depression qi stagnation or depressive heat.

When looked at from this perspective, the menstrual cycle is made up of four (not always equal) segments corresponding to yin, yang, qi and blood. This relationship is shown in the chart below.

Qi, blood, yin and yang
in relation to the menstrual cycle

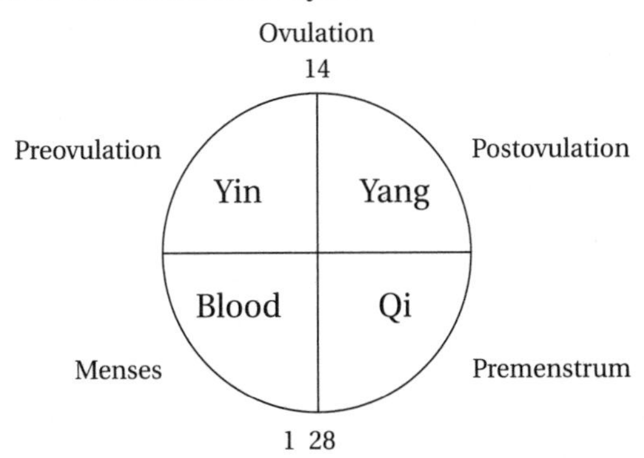

Health problems in women may occur in any of these four phases and may occur for reasons other than the dominant correspondence in that phase. However, when a problem occurs in a woman in any of these four phases, the Chinese medicine practitioner will first investigate to see if the dominant correspondence – yin, yang, qi or blood – is behaving as it should at that time.

AGEING AND DEPRESSION

In Chinese medicine, ageing is seen as a decline in the production and free flow of the qi and blood in both men and women. Typically, first the spleen becomes weak, for instance at around 35 years of age in most women and then, later on, due to the interdependence of the spleen and kidneys, the kidneys become vacuous and weak. As the spleen and kidneys work hand in hand in the production of the qi and blood, this production becomes scantier and scantier. The qi can only keep moving if there is sufficient qi being manufactured to keep propelling it, so this decline in qi production is often accompanied by an inverse rise in signs and symptoms of liver depression and qi stagnation. This is aggravated by the decline in blood production, since blood is necessary to nourish and maintain the liver's coursing and discharge function. In addition, liver function is based on the yang warmth supplied to the liver by the kidneys. The decline and debility of kidney yang, sometimes called the life gate fire, adds to this aggravation of liver depression qi stagnation. Therefore, signs and symptoms associated with liver depression on the one hand and spleen–kidney vacuity on the other all tend to increase past a certain age. Since the heart spirit is an accumulation of qi nourished and kept healthy by the blood, as qi production falls off, the spirit becomes weaker, i.e. less clear or bright. As blood production falls off, the spirit becomes unquiet or restless. Hence, there are many factors that can influence depression in women that relate to the Chinese medical view of the menstrual cycle.

MENOPAUSE AND CHINESE MEDICINE

In women, eventually, the body in its wisdom recognises it is not healthy to try to create qi and blood to nourish and empower the rest of the body at the same time as continuing to menstruate regularly with the loss of blood that that necessarily entails. Therefore, the body initiates a transformation, which, from the Chinese medical point of view, is literally a 'change in life'. The Chinese medical literature does not say exactly how, but at some point the heart ceases sending blood down to collect in the uterus. Just as maturation does not happen all at once, this process is also a gradual one in most women. Therefore, the menses do not just suddenly cease, but menopause is commonly preceded by months or even years of a certain amount of menstrual irregularity. Nevertheless, sooner or later, the heart stops sending blood down to the uterus. Instead, the kidneys are now free to send essence up to accumulate in the heart where it joins with the qi and blood sent up by the spleen and is transformed into spirit.

Thus the woman goes from mother of babies to mother of her tribe, the *femme sage* or wise woman, full of spirit. If this change occurs smoothly, it naturally puts an end to any premenstrual or menopausal depression. There is now more blood available to keep the liver harmonised and functioning correctly and there is more blood to nourish and quiet or calm the heart spirit. Since the spleen and kidneys do not have to create as much blood, they have more energy available to them. They are able to propel the qi more easily through the body, thus keeping it warm, including the liver. All this results in the availability of more yang qi and less qi stagnation.

Unfortunately, the smooth cessation of menstruation is, like all other transformations in the body, dependent on the free flow of liver qi. Since there is no PMS without liver depression qi stagnation, women's menopausal complaints tend to be, both in Chinese theory and in our clinical experience, proportional to the severity of their PMS. In other words, premenstrual and menopausal depression are ultimately not two separate diseases but an unfortunate continuum whose core issue is liver depression qi stagnation. Women with menopausal depression are caught in the change. The change in the flow of qi and blood is not complete. Therefore, the above-described factors that normally make for a more relaxed liver and a calmer, more vigorous heart spirit after menopause do not occur.

We have discussed a good bit of fairly complex Chinese medical theory in the last two chapters. Whilst you may not have understood the technical implications of every point, you will have had the opportunity to see that Chinese medicine is based on an elaborate, sophisticated and, in its own way, logical theory. It is more highly developed than a primitive folk medicine. The more of the above theory you can understand, the more the self-care and preventive techniques we suggest in the following pages will make sense. Chinese medicine is quite different from anything you might be familiar with, so please don't be dismayed if you have to read through the text several times.

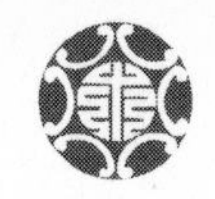

THE CHINESE MEDICAL MECHANISMS OF DEPRESSION

Chinese medicine has a very definite description of the causes and mechanisms of depression. The following description of these mechanisms is from *Zhong Yi Nei Ke Xue (The Study of Chinese Internal Medicine)*. This is the basic textbook on internal medicine used at the Shanghai College of Traditional Chinese Medicine and other provincial Chinese TCM colleges. All the other Chinese medical textbooks we have checked with basically agree with this standard description.

THE DISEASE CAUSES AND MECHANISMS

The onset of depression is due to damage by the emotions. This essentially means emotional turmoil. The liver qi thus becomes depressed and bound, and gradually this leads to disharmony of the qi mechanism of the five viscera. This mainly affects the three viscera of the liver, spleen and heart, causing loss of regulation of the qi and blood. This basic mechanism of liver depression qi stagnation then sets in motion other disease mechanisms, which can be divided into two basic groups: replete conditions where there is an excess of something that is pathological in the body, and vacuity conditions where there is an insufficiency of something in the body necessary for healthy physiology or functioning.

Repletion disease mechanisms

If, because of depression and anger, the smooth flow of the qi is affected, the liver's function will also be affected and the qi will not be properly coursed and discharged throughout the body. If qi depression persists, then over a period of time it may transform into fire. Qi stagnation may also lead to blood stasis. This means that the blood does not move freely but gathers and accumulates like silt in a river. If liver depression 'reaches', i.e. affects, the spleen, if thinking and worry are unresolved or if overwork and fatigue damage the spleen, all these may make the spleen lose its fortification and movement. Since the spleen is in charge of the movement and transformation of body fluids, a lack of spleen fortification and movement may lead to dampness brewing and engendering phlegm.[4] This then leads to qi stagnation and phlegm depression. Since the qi moves and transforms the foods and liquids taken into the stomach, if the qi becomes depressed and does not move, this may give rise to food stagnation. Furthermore, because qi's nature is inherently warm, if qi becomes depressed and accumulates it may transform into depressive heat or fire.

Vacuity disease mechanisms

If there is emotional turmoil or upset, then liver depression may repress the spleen. As the spleen is the source of qi and blood engenderment and transformation, this may result in consumption and damage of the heart qi. The constructive qi and blood are progressively consumed and the heart loses its nourishment, while the spirit loses its treasuring or storage. This is called 'anxiety and depression damaging the spirit' and can lead to a stirring-up of the heart spirit. If such depression persists for a long time with poor nourishment because of decreased eating and drinking, damaging the spleen, then the qi and blood may become insufficient, as there will be an insufficient source for their creation and transformation. In these circumstances, the heart and spleen both become vacuous or depleted. When this spleen vacuity endures, it may

[4] In Chinese medicine, phlegm is nothing other than congealed dampness. Dampness may be congealed into phlegm for any of three reasons: if dampness gathers and collects and is not moved and transformed for a long time, it may congeal into phlegm; if heat stews the juices, it may cook or brew the body fluids into phlegm; cold may freeze or congeal dampness into phlegm.

affect the kidneys, giving rise to kidney–spleen dual vacuity. As we have seen above, if depression endures, it may also transform into fire which easily damages and consumes yin blood. This then affects the kidneys, causing a condition known as 'yin vacuity with fire effulgence'.

MECHANISMS OF DEPRESSION

Therefore, according to Chinese medical theory, depression is basically due to the qi mechanism, which becomes depressed and stagnant as a result of emotional upset. If it persists for many days or if it occurs in someone who is already depleted and weak, for instance due to chronic disease, old age or the menstrual cycle, it can consume and damage the heart qi which is the basis of the spirit. If it goes on longer, it damages and consumes heart blood and spleen qi. If it goes on yet longer, it may also damage kidney yang and/or consume kidney yin. This means that depression of recent onset in relatively young people or those with robust constitutions primarily has to do with liver depression, depressive heat and phlegm fire, while chronic depression or depression in those who are constitutionally weak is a combination of liver depression with vacuity or insufficiencies of heart qi, spleen qi, heart blood, kidney yin and/or kidney yang. Since yin controls yang, if yin is deficient and unable to do this, the result will be vacuity or empty heat, which rises upwards in the body to disturb the spirit in the heart.

The above disease mechanisms may be further aggravated by a number of other factors besides emotional stress and frustration. Whilst a lack of free flow of the emotions may be the primary cause of depression, diet and exercise also play very important roles. For instance, if you consume a lot of fried, fatty, greasy, spicy, or hot, peppery foods, this makes it all the more likely that simple liver depression will transform into depressive heat. If you consume a lot of fatty, greasy foods or eat a lot of dairy products and meat, these damp, phlegmatic foods make the formation of phlegm all the more likely. Eating an excess of sugar and sweets, including fruit juices, or eating a lot of chilled, frozen or uncooked foods, can damage the spleen and tend to cause or aggravate dampness. The spleen may also be damaged by too little exercise, too much work and/or standing too long, although a certain amount of exercise strengthens the spleen, moves the qi and helps course a depressed, stagnant liver. Thus diet and lifestyle play a significant role in both the production and prevention of depression, according to Chinese medicine.

Furthermore, due to the relationships between the five viscera, six bowels, qi, blood and body fluids, the basic disease mechanisms of depression described above may also cause other secondary pathological changes. For example, in the case of the repletion disease mechanisms discussed earlier, it is mentioned that qi stagnation may give rise to blood stasis. This is because the qi moves the blood; if the qi moves, the blood moves and if the qi stops, the blood stops. It is therefore not unusual to find signs and symptoms of blood stasis in people with persistent liver depression qi stagnation (especially women) even though blood stasis per se is not described in the Chinese medical literature as a cause of depression. Also, since the qi moves and transforms the digested food, if there is qi stagnation, it is easy likely for there also to be food stagnation.

Based on our clinical experience in applying this theory to Western patients with depression, liver depression qi stagnation due to emotional stress and frustration may be the single factor that causes a depression. However, in most cases, liver depression qi stagnation combines with and aggravates pre-existing tendencies to imbalances in other viscera and bowels. The specific mechanisms triggered by a failure in the functions of coursing and discharge determine the individual's symptoms of depression, the nature and duration of the depressive episode and the prognosis and outcome of the treatment. Most major depressive episodes involve liver depression qi stagnation as a main component. In dysthymia (low mood) as well as recurrent, chronic and recalcitrant cases of depression, liver depression qi stagnation progresses further to affect the blood and body fluids or occurs on a background of long-standing constitutional insufficiency.

So in Chinese medicine there are likely to be different causes and mechanisms for depression in different people. Some of the causes have to do with mental–emotional causes and reactions. Others have to do with either too much or too little exercise and activity. Some may be due to other diseases in the body. Others are related to age and body type. An incorrect or poor diet may be a contributory factor. Since depression in different people has different underlying causes and disease mechanisms, no one treatment will be effective for everyone. The benefit of Chinese medicine is that individuals can identify their own patterns of depression, and following on from that, identify contributory influences. By correcting these and having the right treatment there may be healing without side-effects from medication.

THE CHINESE MEDICAL TREATMENT OF DEPRESSION

Fundamental to traditional Chinese medicine (TCM) is what is known as treatment based on 'pattern discrimination'. Modern Western medicine bases its treatment on a disease diagnosis. This means that two patients diagnosed as suffering from the same disease will get the same treatment. Whilst TCM does take the patient's disease diagnosis into account, the choice of treatment is not so much based on the disease diagnosis as it is on what is called the patient's pattern. This aspect of Chinese medicine makes it holistic, safe and effective.

In order to explain the difference between a disease and pattern, let us take the symptom of a headache as an example. All headaches by definition must involve some pain in the head. In modern Western medicine and other medical systems that prescribe primarily on the basis of a disease diagnosis, there is likely to be some sort of specific headache medication given. Headache sufferers could, however, be quite different – man or woman, young or old, overweight or thin, for example. The actual symptoms of the headache could also vary – location of pain, left or right side; type of pain, throbbing and continuous or sharp but intermittent, etc. One sufferer could also have the following symptoms: indigestion, a tendency to loose stools, cold feet, red eyes, a dry mouth and desire for cold drinks; another sufferer might have a wet, weeping, crusty skin rash with red borders, a tendency to hay fever, ringing in their ears and dizziness when they stand up. According to both Chinese medicine and modern Western medicine, both people suffer from a headache; however, they also suffer from a whole host of other complaints and may have very different types of headaches and very different constitutions, ages and sex. In Chinese medicine, the patient's pattern is made up from all these other signs and symptoms and further information. In Chinese medicine, the pattern tries to describe the totality of the person as a unique individual. Treatment is designed to rebalance that entire pattern of imbalance as well as address the major complaint, symptom or disease. There is a saying in Chinese medicine: 'One disease, different treatments. Different diseases, same treatment.'

This effectively means that, in Chinese medicine, two patients with the same named disease diagnosis may receive different treatments if their Chinese medical patterns are different, while two patients diagnosed with different named diseases may receive the same treatment if their Chinese medical pattern is the same. The result is that each person is treated individually.

Since every patient gets an individually tailored treatment to restore balance, there are usually no side-effects. Side-effects come from forcing one part of the body to behave while causing an imbalance in some other part. The treatment may have been appropriate to relieve part of the problem but it does not take into account the whole. This is a little like robbing Peter to pay Paul. The fact that Chinese medicine takes many aspects of a person into account in both diagnosis and treatment and looks at the body and mind as a single, unified whole means that a problem is treated without creating further imbalances.

Below is a description of the major Chinese medical patterns seen in patients with the modern Western disease of depression. They are a combination of patterns taken from *Zhong Yi Nei Ke Xue (The Study of Chinese Medicine Internal Medicine)* by Zhang Bo-ying *et al*, and *Xian Dai Nan Zhi Bing Zhong Yi Zhen Liao Xue (A Study of the Chinese Medical Diagnosis and Treatment of Modern, Difficult to Treat Diseases)* by Wu Jun-yu and Bai Yong-bo. Basically, these are the signs and symptoms associated with the disease mechanisms discussed in the previous chapter. Following these signs and symptoms are the treatment principles necessary to redress or correct the imbalance implied in the name of the pattern. These treatment principles tell a person what to do to correct each pattern. Anything that embodies or conforms to those principles will help the patient under discussion, while anything that goes against these principles will aggravate the person's condition.

TREATMENT BASED ON PATTERN DISCRIMINATION – REPLETION PATTERNS

First we shall examine repletion patterns.

Liver depression qi stagnation

Main symptoms

Irritability, a tendency to sigh, premenstrual breast distension and pain, chest oppression and rib-side pain, lower abdominal distension and pain, discomfort in the stomach and epigastrium, diminished appetite, possible delayed menstruation with either scanty or profuse, darkish, stagnant menstrual blood, the menses unable to come easily, a normal or slightly dark tongue with thin, slimy, white fur and a bowstring, fine pulse (see Glossary, page 165). In addition, when there is depression, there is also typically a desire not to see people and not to talk.

Analysis of symptoms

Emotional upset, stress and frustration may damage the liver, resulting in an impairment of its ability to function, particularly in terms of regulating the smooth flow of qi and emotions. This means there is further emotional upset, depression and repression of the emotions. The liver channel traverses the lower abdomen and mixes with the stomach. Then it spreads across the chest and sides of the ribs. If there is liver qi depression and stagnation with lack of smooth flow of the qi mechanism, the qi becomes stagnant and the blood static. The liver network vessels lose their harmony and there is abdominal distension, chest oppression, rib-side pain and even blocked and problematic menstruation in women. If the liver qi attacks the stomach, the stomach loses its harmony and cannot move the food down, resulting in epigastric oppression, belching, burping, lack of appetite and, in some cases, even nausea and vomiting. If the liver assails the spleen, this leads to abdominal distension and affects defecation. The thin, slimy tongue fur and the bowstring pulse are signs of liver–stomach disharmony from an Oriental medical perspective.

Treatment principles
Course the liver, rectify the qi and resolve depression.

Liver depression transforms heat

Main symptoms
The signs and symptoms are the same as for liver depression qi stagnation, with the following differences. Firstly, the patient is not just irritable, they are downright angry. Secondly, there is a bitter taste in their mouth in the mornings when they wake. Thirdly, there is a red tongue with yellow fur and a bowstring, rapid pulse. Other symptoms may include tinnitus, headache, red eyes, dry mouth, dry, bound, constipated stools, violent outbursts of anger, swearing, shouting and physically throwing or destroying things.

Analysis of symptoms
Qi depression has transformed into fire either because it was long-lasting or because it was severe. The nature of fire is to flare upwards. In this case it follows the liver vessels and moves upwards. This results in headache, red eyes and tinnitus. If liver fire attacks the stomach, the stomach and intestines will have heat. The mouth will be dry and may have a bitter taste in it, whilst the stools are constipated and bound.

Emotional tension, agitation, quick temper, a red tongue with yellow fur and a bowstring, rapid pulse are all signs of liver fire.

Treatment principles

Course the liver, rectify the qi, clear heat and resolve depression.

Liver blood stasis and stagnation

Main symptoms

Emotional depression, heart vexation and agitation, suicidal thoughts, a dark, dusky facial complexion, rib-side and flank distension and pain, possible amenorrhoea (absence of periods) or painful menstruation in women, a dark, purplish tongue, possibly showing small spots or bumps, white fur and a deep, bowstring or choppy pulse.

Analysis of symptoms

If liver depression persists or is very severe, the qi may fail to move the blood. The blood, therefore, becomes static due to the qi being stagnant. Here we have a combination of liver depression qi stagnation signs and symptoms, such as the rib-side distension and bowstring pulse, along with blood stasis symptoms, such as lower abdominal or menstrual pain, a purple tongue or a choppy pulse.

Treatment principles

Course the liver and move the qi, quicken the blood and transform stasis.

Phlegm dampness obstruction and stagnation

Main symptoms

Discomfort within the throat as if there were something obstructing and blocking the throat that can neither be swallowed down or spat out, oppression within the chest, possible simultaneous rib-side pain, slimy, white tongue fur and a bowstring, slippery pulse.

Analysis of symptoms

If liver depression assails the spleen and the spleen movement loses its fortification, then dampness will be created and this may gather into phlegm. Phlegm and qi then become depressed and bound in the chest and above the diaphragm. The discomfort within the throat, as if there were something blocking and obstructing it, is due to a phlegm and qi blockage. It is called 'plum stone qi' because the Chinese liken this sensation to having a plum stone stuck in your throat. If qi loses its soothing, then there is oppression within the chest. The rib-sides are the place where the liver channel spreads across. If the channels and network vessels of the liver become depressed and stagnant, then there is rib-side pain. The slimy, white tongue fur and the bowstring, slippery pulse are symptoms of liver depression mixed with phlegm dampness.

Treatment principles

Transform phlegm, free the qi and resolve depression.

Phlegm fire harassing the spirit

Main symptoms

Insomnia, a heavy, full, stuffy or tight feeling in the head, excessive or profuse phlegm, chest oppression, aversion to food, burping and belching, acid regurgitation, possible nausea, heart vexation, a bitter taste in the mouth, vertigo and dizziness, slimy, yellow tongue fur and a slippery, rapid, possibly also bowstring pulse. In cases of depression, the person will feel profoundly apathetic and tired, yet restless and anxious, or may alternate between one and the other.

Analysis of symptoms

Basically, this pattern is the same as the previous one except for the addition of heat or fire. The manifestations of this heat are the heart vexation, agitation insomnia, the bitter taste in the mouth, the yellow tongue fur and the rapid pulse.

Treatment principles
Transform phlegm and clear heat, harmonise the stomach and quiet the spirit.

TREATMENT BASED ON PATTERN DISCRIMINATION – VACUITY PATTERNS

Other symptom patterns may be described as vacuity patterns.

Anxiety and worry harassing the heart spirit

Main symptoms
Mental–emotional abstraction, restlessness, sorrow and anxiety, a tendency to crying, frequent yawning, a pale tongue with thin, white fur and a bowstring, fine pulse.

Analysis of symptoms
If anxiety and depression are not resolved, the heart qi is consumed and damaged and the qi and blood become depleted and unable to nourish the heart spirit. One sees mental–emotional abstraction and restlessness. The pale tongue with thin, white fur and the bowstring, fine pulse are signs of qi depression and blood vacuity.

Treatment principles
Nourish the heart and quiet the spirit.

Heart–spleen dual vacuity

Main symptoms
Excessive thinking with a tendency to worry, heart palpitations, gall bladder timidity, poor sleep, poor memory, a lustreless facial complexion, dizziness, lassitude of the spirit, devitalised eating and drinking, a pale tongue and a fine, weak pulse. In depressed patients exhibiting this pattern, there is pronounced confusion, lack of concentration, lack of strength in the arms and legs and severe fatigue.

Analysis of symptoms

If the heart is taxed by thinking and worry, the heart and spleen may both become vacuous. The heart thus loses its nourishment, and one sees heart palpitations, timidity, poor sleep and poor memory. The spleen and stomach are the source of the engenderment and transformation of the qi and blood. If the spleen does not fortify and move, then the appetite is diminished and the source of qi and blood is insufficient. One sees a lustreless facial complexion, dizziness, lassitude of the spirit, fatigue, lack of strength, a pale tongue and a fine, weak pulse.

Treatment principles

Fortify the spleen and nourish the heart, boost the qi and supplement the blood.

Spleen–kidney yang vacuity

Main symptoms

Emotional listlessness and depression, a desire to lie down and be still, heart vexation, fright and fear, heart palpitations and loss of sleep, a sombre white facial complexion, impotence in men or involuntary seminal emission, clear, watery vaginal discharge in women, decreased or absent libido in both men and women, lower back soreness, cold feet, a fat, pale tongue, possibly with teeth marks on its edges and white fur, and a deep, fine pulse.

Analysis of symptoms

If spleen qi vacuity endures or worsens and reaches the kidneys, kidney yang may also become vacuous and insufficient. If this happens, the signs and symptoms of qi vacuity are even more pronounced, such as a desire to lie down and not move, plus there are symptoms of specifically kidney yang vacuity, such as lack of libido, lower back soreness and cold feet. Many women exhibit this pattern as they enter their perimenopausal years.

Treatment principles

Warm the kidneys and fortify the spleen, invigorate yang and boost the qi.

Yin vacuity with fire effulgence

Main symptoms

Vertigo and dizziness, heart palpitations, poor sleep, heart vexation, quick temper, possible involuntary seminal emission in men, lower back soreness, menstrual irregularities in women, a red tongue and a bowstring, fine and rapid pulse. In patients with depression, there is much anxiety, vexation and agitation and restlessness.

Analysis of symptoms

If kidney yin is insufficient and the blood and body fluids are consumed by heat, depleted yin may not be able to control yang and hence yang floats upwards. One may see vertigo, dizziness and quick temper. If there is yin and blood depletion and consumption, then the heart spirit loses its nourishment. In addition, yin vacuity gives rise to heat and vacuity heat harasses the spirit. This leads to heart palpitations, poor sleep, anxiety and agitation. If kidney yin is insufficient, then the lower back mansion loses its nourishment and this leads to low back soreness. With this situation of yin vacuity combined with fire effulgence, the effulgent fire harasses and stirs the essence chamber. Hence the essence is not secured and there is seminal emission. If the liver and kidneys lose their nourishment, the *chong* and *ren*, two vessels that in Chinese medicine are believed to control menstruation and that are related to the liver and kidneys respectively, will be unregulated. This can result in menstrual irregularities. The red tongue and bowstring, fine, rapid pulse are both signs of yin vacuity.

Treatment principles

Enrich yin and clear heat, settle the heart and quiet the spirit.

THE REAL DEAL

Although textbook discriminations such as the one above make it seem as if all the practitioner has to do is match up their patient's symptoms with one of the aforementioned patterns and then prescribe the recommended guiding formula, in actual clinical practice, one usually encounters combinations of the above discrete patterns and their related disease mechanisms or progressions. For instance, liver depression transforming heat may be complicated by spleen qi and heart blood vacuity or by spleen qi and kidney yang vacuity. This in turn may also be complicated by phlegm or blood stasis. Likewise, yin vacuity with fire effulgence may be complicated by liver depression and spleen qi vacuity, liver depression and blood stasis or liver depression and phlegm. In particular, liver depression and spleen vacuity go hand in hand in clinical practice. Rarely in our clinical experience do you see one without the other, especially in Westerners (relating to lifestyle and diet). This means that attention to and remedy of the causes and mechanisms of liver depression qi stagnation and spleen qi vacuity are almost always useful when dealing with depression. *Nei Jing (The Inner Classic)*, the 'bible' of Chinese medicine says, 'If the liver is diseased, first treat the spleen.' Once you have these two pivotal patterns, then all the rest of the patterns described above may easily evolve. In chronic, recurrent depression and dysthymia, there is usually long-standing phlegm obstruction, blood stasis, extreme insufficiency of qi and blood or a combination of these elements. In bipolar disorder or manic depression, there is always some sort of heat involved which gives rise to the mania. The three patterns, all involving heat, that Wu and Bai describe for the manic part of bipolar disorder are liver fire internally harassing, liver–gall bladder depressive heat and exuberant heat damaging yin.

HOW THIS SYSTEM WORKS IN REAL LIFE

Using all the above information on the theory of Chinese medicine and the patterns and their mechanisms of depression, let's see how a Chinese medicine practitioner makes this system work in real life.

CASE STUDY

Take Joan, for example, whom we introduced at the beginning of this book. She has experienced depression on and off since she was about 13. In this most recent episode, she has been feeling depressed for a couple of months. She feels increasingly irritable and frustrated. She can't control her feelings, cries frequently and wants only to be alone, feeling unmotivated and tired all the time. She wants to sleep constantly but has trouble falling asleep. Once she does fall asleep, her sleep is disturbed by intense dreams. Joan is 24 years old. She is slightly overweight, looks a bit puffy, but her musculature feels strong. She has trouble losing weight, eats constantly to calm herself down and says she has gained a lot of weight lately. She feels bloated, burps a lot and craves sweets. When she eats dairy products, eggs, sugar or fatty foods, her fatigue increases and she produces more mucus. Joan also says she feels worried, has trouble focusing and feels overwhelmed by details. She is anxious, agitated and can't think clearly. Since she gets annoyed so easily, she feels bad about herself and sometimes guilty.

Like many women, Joan's depression gets worse before her period. Premenstrually, she also gets abdominal distension, craves sweets and has an increased appetite. Her breasts become sore and painful, especially the nipples. Her emotions fluctuate constantly and she feels extremely irritable, lashing out at the people around her. Her periods have always been irregular, sometimes coming early, sometimes late. She also bleeds excessively once her period does come, sometimes for more than a week. Her blood flow is darker at the beginning and mixed with blood clots. It flows intermittently, stopping and starting.

In addition, her tongue appears puffy, a bit redder than normal, especially the sides and tip. It trembles, has a deep crack in the centre and white-yellowish fur which is thicker towards the back. Her pulse is bowstring and rather slippery. It also feels soggy over her wrist bone on the right side.

How a Chinese medicine practitioner analyses Joan's symptoms

Joan's irritability, frustration, wanting to be alone, burping, premenstrual breast distension and her bowstring pulse all indicate liver depression qi stagnation. Her constant hunger, thirst, dry mouth and red tongue indicate that this stagnation has transformed into heat, which is affecting the stomach. This is corroborated by the especially sensitive and sore nipples premenstrually, a strong sign of depressive heat in the liver. Her agitation, restlessness, insomnia and dream-disturbed sleep indicate that this heat is also disturbing the spirit residing in the heart. Her weight gain, abdominal distension after meals, fatigue and facial oedema (puffiness) as well as the soggy pulse on her right wrist, all indicate spleen vacuity or weakness. This is further indicated by increased fatigue when she eats foods that damage the spleen and generate dampness. As she has a weak spleen, dampness and phlegm have accumulated, which then obstruct the free flow of qi all the more. When her menses come late, this is because of the liver depression qi stagnation. Her early periods and heavy menstrual bleeding are probably a combination of depressive heat forcing the blood to run frenetically outside its channels, and spleen qi vacuity failing to hold the blood within its channels. Based on the clots in her menstruate, there may even be some blood stasis due to long-term qi stagnation.

Due to Joan's constitutional body type, it is likely that her spleen vacuity is, at least in part, constitutional. Everyone has constitutional differences, including the relative strengths and weaknesses of the viscera and bowels. Some people are born with a weaker spleen than others. In Joan's case, her depressive episodes have historically been precipitated by psychosocial stress factors. In other words, spleen depletion or vacuity on its own, even with dampness and phlegm, is not enough to trigger a depressive episode in Joan. It is only when it is compounded by liver depression qi stagnation, which then leads to further weakening of the spleen, that the end result is a depressive episode. Once a depressive episode starts, Joan's diet and behaviour can either keep it going or lighten it and bring it to an end. Joan's depression is also intimately connected with her menstrual and premenstrual complaints. The improvement of the one would simultaneously improve the other, according to Chinese medicine.

When all this information is put together, the Chinese medicine practitioner knows that there is liver depression with depressive heat harassing above, spleen vacuity with phlegm and dampness gumming up the works and maybe an element of blood stasis. Whether or not this last element exists is yet to be conclusively decided but may become clear once treatment has been initiated.

How a Chinese medicine practitioner treats Joan's depression

Once a practitioner of Chinese medicine knows the patient's pattern discrimination, the next step is to formulate the appropriate treatment in order to rebalance the problems. If liver depression transforming heat is decided on as the main pattern, then the treatment principles are to course the liver and rectify the qi, clear heat and resolve depression. If it is decided that there is spleen vacuity secondarily, then the next principles are to fortify the spleen and boost the qi. If this spleen vacuity has given rise to phlegm and dampness, then the principles of eliminating dampness and transforming phlegm would be added.

One of the features of Chinese medicine is that once the practitioner has stated the treatment principles, it is highly likely that any treatment or change in lifestyle that works to accomplish these principles will be beneficial for the patient. The Chinese medicine practitioner has several treatment options in addition to acupuncture and Chinese herbal medicinals, recommendations may also be given regarding diet and lifestyle. The practitioner may be able to advise the patient on many aspects of their life according to what will be beneficial for them based on a Chinese medicine pattern diagnosis.

In Chinese medicine one of the main treatment modalities is the prescribing of Chinese 'herbal' medicinals.[5] A prescription for Joan would be put together as follows: since the treatment principles stated for Joan were to course the liver and rectify the qi, clear heat and resolve depression, and as the liver depression is complicating a pattern of spleen vacuity with dampness and phlegm, the Chinese herbalist would select their guiding formula from the 'harmonising the liver and spleen' category of formulae. Depending on the textbook, there are 22–28 main categories of formulae in Chinese medicine, each category correlated to a main treatment principle. The category of harmonising the liver and spleen is part of a broader category of harmonising formulae which are used to treat patterns that involve complex processes in different levels of the body and different organs, as well as the simultaneous presence of hot and cold.

---

[5] The world 'herbal' is in quotation marks since Chinese medicine is not entirely herbal. Herbs are medicinals made from parts of plants, their roots, bark, stems, leaves, flowers, etc. Chinese medicinals are mostly herbal in nature. However, a percentage of Chinese medicinals also come from the animal and mineral realms. Thus not all Chinese medicinals are, strictly speaking, herbs.

Under this category of formulae, there is one that is well known for addressing several of the treatment principles we have decided to be appropriate for Joan, *Xiao Chao Hu Tang* (Minor Bupleurum Combination/Decoction). This formula can be used for a wide variety of complaints characterised, on the one hand, by liver depression qi stagnation with the presence of heat and, on the other hand, by spleen vacuity giving rise to dampness and phlegm. The Chinese herbalist might then modify this prescription to clear even more heat, boost the qi more, eliminate dampness or transform phlegm more or to address her menstrual complaints more effectively.

If the formula was modified from its textbook or standard form in order to better suit a patient's needs, the final formula would be called *Xiao Chai Hu Tang Jia Wei* (Minor Bupleurum Decoction with Added Flavours i.e. ingredients). The standard formula comprises:

Radix Bupleuri *(Chai Hu)*
Radix Panacis Ginseng *(Ren Shen)*
Radix Scutellariae Baicalensis *(Huang Qin)*
Rhizoma Pinelliae Ternatae *(Ban Xia)*
Uncooked Rhizoma Zingiberis *(Sheng Jiang)*
Mix-fried Radix Glycyrrhizae *(Gan Cao)*
Fructus Zizyphi Jujubae *(Da Zao)*

The action of the medicinals is as follows: Bupleurum courses the liver and rectifies the qi while scattering internal heat through diaphoresis (sweating). Ginseng is a tonic which fortifies the spleen and supplements the qi of the entire organism. It also quiets the spirit. Scutellaria clears heat from the lungs and stomach (manifested as uncontrolled crying and excessive appetite) as well as from the liver and heart. Pinellia harmonises the stomach. It also transforms phlegm and eliminates dampness via the spleen's movement and transformation. Uncooked or fresh ginger (zingiberis) assists pinellia in all of these functions and promotes the movement of qi. Glycyrrhiza or liquorice supplements the spleen and heart. It also helps harmonise all the other ingredients in the formula and prevents them from having unwanted side-effects. Zizyphus Jujube or red dates supplement the spleen and nourish the heart. In this formula, they assist ginseng and liquorice.

Some of the medicinals that might be added in order to modify this formula to Joan's condition and needs are Cortex Albizziae Julibrissinis *(He Huan Pi)* to calm her spirit – this herb is used for insomnia and irritability due to qi stagnation; Radix Polygalae Tenuifoliae *(Yuan Zhi)*, which both calms the spirit and transforms phlegm – it is very helpful in cases of depression characterised by excessive brooding and disorientation combined with constrained emotions; and Rhizoma Acori Graminei *(Shi Chang Pu)*, an aromatic substance which transforms phlegm and 'opens the orifices', and is used when phlegm blocks and prevents the clear yang of consciousness. As we saw in the section describing the continuum of phlegm dampness obstruction and stagnation patterns, phlegm confounding the orifices of the heart may cause lassitude of the spirit, lack of clarity of thought, confusion and excessive rumination.

Usually, a formula such as this when used to treat depression would be taken two to three times each day. The herbs would be soaked in water and then boiled into a very strong 'tea' for 30–45 minutes. Each week, the practitioner would check with Joan to see how she was doing and if any modifications to her formula were needed. Remember, the practitioner of Chinese medicine wants to heal without causing any side-effects. If the formula does cause any unwanted effects, then the practitioner will add and subtract ingredients until the herbs achieve the desired result with no unwanted effects.

The ingredients in this formula may also be taken as a dried, powdered extract. Such extracts are manufactured by several Taiwanese and Japanese companies. Although such extracts are not, in our experience, always as powerful as the freshly decocted teas, they are easier to take. Many standard formulae also come as ready-made pills which cannot be modified. If their ingredients match the individual patient's requirements, then they can be very beneficial. If the formula needs modifications, then teas or powders whose individual ingredients can be added and subtracted are better.

In exactly the same way, the practitioner of Chinese medicine could create an individual acupuncture treatment plan and an accompanying dietary and lifestyle plan. These treatments will be discussed later on in the book. In a woman of Joan's age with her Chinese pattern discrimination, either Chinese herbal medicine alone, acupuncture alone or a combination of the two supported by the proper diet and lifestyle would probably eliminate, or at the very least diminish, her depression within two to three weeks. Often there is an improvement after the first day of taking a full dose of the herbs. The herbs, however, do not work in the same way as antidepressants. They act to restore balance and harmony to the yin and yang of the body and in so doing may have many other beneficial effects.

CHINESE HERBAL MEDICINE AND DEPRESSION

As we have seen from Joan's case, there is no single Chinese 'antidepression herb' or even an 'antidepression formula' that would suit all sufferers of depression. Chinese medicinals are individually prescribed based on a person's pattern discrimination, not on a disease diagnosis like depression. Patients often come to practitioners of Chinese medicine saying, 'A friend told me that *Xiao Yao Wan* (Free and Easy Pills, a common Chinese over-the-counter medication) is good for depression. Yet when I tried it, it didn't work.' This is because *Xiao Yao Wan* is meant to treat a specific pattern of depression, not depression per se. If you exhibit that pattern, then this formula will work. If you do not have signs and symptoms of that pattern, it won't.

As most people's depression is a combination of different Chinese patterns and disease mechanisms, a practitioner of Chinese medicine never treats depression with a single herb given all on its own. Chinese herbal medicine is based on rebalancing patterns, and patterns in real-life patients almost always have more than a single element. So herbs are almost always prescribed in multi-ingredient formulae. Such formulae may have anywhere from four to 18 or more ingredients. If a practitioner of Chinese medicine reads a prescription given by another practitioner, they will be able to tell not only what the patient's pattern discrimination was but also what the likely signs and symptoms were. In creating a herbal formula, the practitioner of Chinese medicine does not just combine several herbs which are reputed to be 'good for depression'. Rather, a formula is carefully crafted with ingredients to rebalance every aspect of the patient's body–mind.

GETTING THE RIGHT HERBAL MEDICINE TREATMENT FOR YOURSELF

Chinese herbal medicine has become increasingly popular in the West, particularly in the UK. It does, however, require a high level of study as it is quite complex, and we strongly recommend that you seek professional advice. As well as the signs and symptoms of an illness, a practitioner of Chinese medicine will take into account additional information, such as tongue and pulse diagnosis, in order to decide which herbs are appropriate. These skills require experience and training and are beyond the scope of this book. This means that the self-prescribing of Chinese herbs is really not something for the layperson to attempt, especially if unsupervised. As a layperson it is unlikely that you will be able to obtain Chinese herbs without a prescription from a qualified practitioner in the UK, as reputable suppliers will not generally sell directly to the public. Chinese herbal medicines can be very powerful; just as they have the power to heal, they can also do damage if incorrectly used. Later, we will give suggestions on how to find a qualified professional Chinese medical practitioner.

The remainder of this chapter will focus on what are commonly known as Chinese herbal patent remedies or 'patents'. These are herbal remedies that have been used for many years, often for centuries, and have therefore earned a tried and tested track record for treating illness. In some countries they may be available over the counter in a health food shop or Chinese herb specialist shop but we strongly recommend that you do not take them unsupervised. We have included them here as they demonstrate how Chinese herbal medicine treats depression. Even an individually tailored herbal medicine prescription will often include the herbs presented in these formulae.

The patents we have included can be used to treat the key or basic patterns associated with depression we discussed earlier. These are:

Liver depression qi stagnation
Liver depression transforms heat
Liver blood stasis and stagnation
Phlegm dampness obstruction and stagnation
Phlegm fire harassing the spirit
Anxiety and worry harassing the heart spirit
Heart–spleen dual vacuity
Spleen–kidney yang vacuity
Yin vacuity with fire effulgence

If you are able to identify your main pattern, then it is likely that a herbal prescription could include some of the herbs detailed in the relevant patent formula for that pattern.

***Xiao Yao Wan* (also spelt *Hsiao Yao Wan*)**

Xiao Yao Wan is one of the most commonly prescribed Chinese herbal formulae. Its Chinese name has been translated as Free and Easy Pills, Rambling Pills, Relaxed Wanderer Pills and several other versions of this same idea of promoting a free, smooth and more relaxed flow.

The ingredients in this formula are:

Radix Bupleuri *(Chai Hu)*
Radix Angelicae Sinensis *(Dang Gui)*
Radix Albus Paeoniae Lactiflorae *(Bai Shao)*
Rhizoma Atractylodis Macrocephalae *(Bai Zhu)*
Sclerotium Poriae Cocos *(Fu Ling)*
Mix-fried Radix Glycyrrhizae *(Gan Cao)*
Herba Menthae Haplocalycis *(Bo He)*
Uncooked Rhizoma Zingiberis *(Sheng Jiang)*

This formula treats the pattern of liver depression qi stagnation complicated by blood vacuity and spleen weakness, with possible dampness as well. Bupleurum courses the liver and rectifies the qi. It is aided in this by Herba Menthae Haplocalycis (mint). Dang Gui and Radix Albus Paeoniae Lactiflorae (white peony) nourish the blood and soften and harmonise the liver. Rhizoma Atractylodis

Macrocephalae (atractylodes) and Sclerotium Poriae Cocos (poria) fortify the spleen and eliminate dampness. Mix-fried liquorice aids these two in fortifying the spleen and supplementing the liver, while uncooked ginger aids in both promoting and regulating the qi flow and eliminating dampness.

When depression presents with the signs and symptoms of liver depression, spleen qi vacuity and an element of blood vacuity, this formula can be very effective. If it is not the correct treatment then you may experience some side-effects, which could include nervousness, irritability, a dry mouth, increased thirst and red, dry eyes. This means that this formula is not right for you. Although it may be doing you some good, it is also causing some harm. Remember, Chinese medicine is meant to cure without side-effects and as long as the prescription matches your pattern there will not be any.

Dan Zhi Xiao Yao Wan

Dan Zhi Xiao Yao Wan (Moutan and Gardenia Rambling Pills) is a modification of the above formula that also comes as a patent medicine in the form of pills. When marketed as a dried, powdered extract, this formula is called Bupleurum and Peony Formula. It is meant to treat the pattern of liver depression transforming into heat with spleen vacuity and possible blood vacuity and/or dampness. The ingredients in this formula are the same as above except that two other herbs are added:

Cortex Radicis Moutan *(Dan Pi)*
Fructus Gardeniae Jasminoidis *(Shan Zhi Zi)*

These two ingredients clear heat and resolve depression. In addition, Cortex Radicis Moutan (moutan) quickens the blood and dispels stasis and is good at clearing heat specifically from the blood. Some practitioners prefer to take out uncooked ginger and mint, while other leave these two ingredients in.

Basically, the signs and symptoms of the pattern for which this formula is designed are the same as those for *Xiao Yao Wan* above, plus signs and symptoms of depressive heat. These might include a reddish tongue with slightly yellow fur, a bowstring and rapid pulse, a bitter taste in the mouth and increased irritability.

Chai Hu Jia Long Gu Mu Li Wan

Chai Hu Jia Long Gu Mu Li Wan (Bupleurum, Dragon Bone and Oyster Shell Pills) is the pill form of a formula which has been used in China and other Asian countries for 1,700 years. It is for the treatment of liver depression/depressive heat and spleen vacuity causing mental–emotional anxiety, unrest, insomnia and heart palpitations. Its ingredients include:

Radix Bupleuri *(Chai Hu)*
Radix Panacis Ginseng *(Ren Shen)*
Rhizoma Pinelliae Ternatae *(Ban Xia)*
Sclerotium Poriae Cocos *(Fu Ling)*
Ramulus Cinnamomi Cassiae *(Gui Zhi)*
Radix Scutellariae Baicalensis *(Huang Qin)*
Fructus Zizyphi Jujubae *(Da Zao)*
Os Draconis *(Long Gu)*
Concha Ostreae *(Mu Li)*
Dry Rhizoma Zingiberis *(Gan Jiang)*
Radix Et Rhizoma Rhei *(Da Huang)*

As this formula contains rhubarb (*Da Huang*), it is especially effective for those suffering from constipation. Rhubarb is a strong purgative and if it causes diarrhoea, its use should be immediately discontinued and your practitioner should be informed.

Chai Hu Shu Gan Wan

Chai Hu Shu Gan Wan means Bupleurum Soothe the Liver Pills. They treat liver depression qi stagnation, the main mechanism of most people's depression. These pills course the liver and rectify the qi, resolve depression and loosen the chest. Their ingredients consist of:

Radix Bupleuri *(Chai Hu)*
Radix Albus Paeoniae Lactiflorae *(Bai Shao)*
Rhizoma Cyperi Rotundi *(Xiang Fu)*
Fructus Citri Aurantii *(Zhi Ke)*
Radix Ligustici Wallichii *(Chuan Xiong)*
Radix Glycyrrhizae *(Gan Cao)*

Unlike the preceding formulae, this one does not contain any ingredients that fortify the spleen and supplement the qi. It is completely focused on moving and rectifying the qi.

Da Chai Hu Wan

Meaning Great Bupleurum Pills, this formula is for rather severe liver depression of recent onset or in a robust individual with a tendency to constipation. It courses the liver and rectifies the qi, clears heat and frees the flow of the stools. Its ingredients consist of:

Radix Bupleuri *(Chai Hu)*
Rhizoma Pinelliae Ternatae *(Ban Xia)*
Radix Scutellariae Baicalensis *(Huang Qin)*
Fructus Citri Aurantii *(Zhi Ke)*
Radix Albus Paeoniae Lactiflorae *(Bai Shao)*
Dry Rhizoma Zingiberis *(Gan Jiang)*
Fructus Zizyphi Jujubae *(Da Zao)*
Radix Et Rhizoma Rhei *(Da Huang)*

Like Bupleurum, Dragon Bone and Oyster Shell Pills (see page 73), because this formula contains rhubarb (*Da Huang*), it is especially useful for those with constipation with dry, hard, bound stools.

Xiao Chai Hu Wan

If *Da Chai Hu Wan* means Great Bupleurum Pills, then *Xiao Chai Hu Wan* means Small or Minor Bupleurum Pills. This formula is also for liver depression/depressive heat. It is indicated for those with concomitant spleen vacuity and no constipation. In fact, it is a good formula for those with a tendency to soft or loose stools. This is the pill formula of the prescription given to Joan in the preceding chapter. It is the most commonly prescribed Chinese herbal formula in the world with a wide range of indications. It is called a harmonising formula since it harmonises the inside and outside of the body, the liver and spleen, the spleen and stomach and the stomach and intestines. Its ingredients consist of:

Radix Bupleuri *(Chai Hu)*
Rhizoma Pinelliae Ternatae *(Ban Xia)*
Radix Codonopsitis Pilosulae *(Dang Shen)*
Radix Scutellariae Baicalensis *(Huang Qin)*
Fructus Zizyphi Jujubae *(Da Zao)*
Radix Glycyrrhizae *(Gan Cao)*
Dry Rhizoma Zingiberis *(Gan Jiang)*

Shu Gan Wan

The name of this formula means Soothe the Liver Pills. In English, these pills are erroneously identified as Hepatic Tonic Pills. They primarily course the liver and rectify the qi. They are especially recommended when stagnant qi affects digestion and is accompanied by pain and distension in the upper abdomen and below the ribs. Their ingredients are:

Fructus Meliae Toosendan *(Chuan Lian Zi)*
Rhizoma Curcumae Longae *(Jiang Huang)*
Lignum Aquilariae Agallochae *(Chen Xiang)*
Rhizoma Corydalis Yanhusuo *(Yan Hu Suo)*
Radix Auklandiae Lappae *(Mu Xiang)*
Semen Myrsticae Fragrantis *(Rou Kou)*
Radix Albus Paeoniae Lactiflorae *(Bai Shao)*
Sclerotium Poriae Cocos *(Fu Ling)*
Fructus Citri Aurantii *(Zhi Ke)*

Pericarpium Citri Reticulatae *(Chen Pi)*
Fructus Amomi *(Sha Ren)*
Cortex Magnoliae Officinalis *(Huo Po)*

A condensed version of the same formula is sold as *Shu Kan Wan,* and moves liver depression qi stagnation more effectively. It deletes Fructus Meliae Toosendan and Sclerotium Poriae Cocos and adds eight additional herbs:

Rhizoma Cyperi Rotundi *(Xiang Fu)*
Radix Glycyrrhizae *(Gan Cao)*
Cortex Radicis Moutan *(Dan Pi)*
Radix Bupleuri *(Chai Hu)*
Fructus Citri Sacrodactylis *(Fo Shou)*
Pericarpium Citri Reticulatae Viride *(Qing Pi)*
Fructus Citri Medicae *(Xiang Yuan)*
Lignum Santalli Albi *(Tan Xiang)*

Mu Xiang Shun Qi Wan

The name of this formula translates as Auklandia Normalise the Qi Pills. It courses the liver and rectifies the qi. It is also recommended in cases of qi stagnation affecting the digestion and causing food stagnation. It relieves abdominal pain, boosts the stomach and disperses food accumulation. It is used to treat feelings of fullness in the chest, diaphragm and hypochondrium. Its ingredients are:

Radix Auklandia Lappae *(Mu Xiang)*
Semen Myrsticae Fragrantis *(Dou Kou)*
Rhizoma Atractylodis *(Cang Zhu)*
Uncooked Rhizoma Zingiberis *(Sheng Jiang)*
Pericarpium Citri Reticulatae Viride *(Qing Pi)*
Pericarpium Citri Reticulatae *(Chen Pi)*
Sclerotium Poriae Cocos *(Fu Ling)*
Radix Bupleuri *(Chai Hu)*
Cortex Magnoliae Officinalis *(Hou Po)*
Semen Arecae Catechu *(Bing Lang)*

Fructus Citri Aurantii *(Zhi Ke)*
Radix Linderae Strychnifoliae *(Wu Yao)*
Semen Raphani Sativi *(Lai Fu Zi)*
Fructus Crataegi *(Shan Zha)*
Massa Medica Fermentata *(Shen Qu)*
Fructus Germinatus Hordei Vulgaris *(Mai Ya)*
Radix Glycyrrhizae *(Gan Cao)*

Gan Mai Da Zao Wan

The name of these pills translates as Liquorice, Wheat and Red Dates Pills. This formula is specifically for the pattern of depression known as depression and anxiety harassing the heart. This is a combination of liver depression and heart qi vacuity resulting in restlessness and agitation, alternating tendencies to euphoria and tears and the possibility of night sweats. This small formula can be added to a number of other formulae when either mood swings or night sweats complicate other conditions. The ingredients in this formula are:

Fructus Levis Tritici Aestivi *(Fu Xiao Mai)*
Radix Glycyrrhizae *(Gan Cao)*
Fructus Zizyphi Jujubae *(Da Zao)*
Bulbus Lilii *(Bai He)*
Cortex Albizziae Julibrissinis *(He Huan Pi)*
Radix Polygoni Multiflori *(He Shou Wu)*
Sclerotium Poriae Cocos *(Fu Ling)*

This formula can be especially effective for women's premenstrual and perimenopausal depression and anxiety. If there are night sweats it may be extremely beneficial. One of the ingredients contained in this formula is liquorice, which can raise the blood pressure. It may therefore not be suitable for someone with high blood pressure. However, most women with this condition tend to have lower than normal blood pressure.

An Shen Yang Xin Cha

Marketed under the English name Shen Classic Tea, these prepackaged tea bags are meant for heart qi and blood vacuity with an element of liver depression. They can be drunk as a daily beverage for those with mental–emotional restlessness and anxiety, insomnia and heart palpitations due to heart qi and blood vacuity. They are not meant for these same conditions when due to pathological heat or phlegm. Their ingredients consist of:

Folium Mori Albi *(Sang Ye)*
Sclerotium Poriae Cocos *(Fu Ling)*
Radix Polygoni Multiflori *(He Shou Wu)*
Radix Salviae Miltiorrhizae *(Dan Shen)*
Radix Polygalae Tenuifoliae *(Yuan Zhi)*

***Gui Pi Wan* (also spelt *Kuei Pi Wan*)**

Gui means to return or restore, *pi* means the spleen and *wan* means pills. Therefore, the name of these pills means Restore the Spleen Pills. When marketed as a dried, powdered extract, this formula is called Ginseng and Longan Combination. However, these pills not only supplement the spleen qi but also nourish heart blood and calm the heart spirit. They are the textbook guiding formula for the pattern of heart–spleen dual vacuity. In this case, there are symptoms of spleen qi vacuity, such as fatigue, poor appetite and cold hands and feet plus symptoms of heart blood vacuity, such as a pale tongue, heart palpitations and insomnia. This is also the standard formula for treating heavy or abnormal bleeding due to the spleen not containing and restraining the blood within its vessels. Therefore, this patent medicine can be combined with *Xiao Yao San* when there is liver depression qi stagnation complicated by heart blood and spleen qi vacuity. Its ingredients are:

Radix Astragali Membranacei *(Huang Qi)*
Radix Codonopsitis Pilosulae *(Dang Shen)*

Rhizoma Atractylodis Macrocephalae *(Bai Zhu)*
Sclerotium Pararadicis Poriae Cocos *(Fu Shen)*
Mix-fried Radix Glycyrrhizae *(Gan Cao)*
Radix Angelicae Sinensis *(Dang Gui)*
Semen Zizyphi Spinosae *(Suan Zao Ren)*
Arillus Euphoriae Longanae *(Long Yan Rou)*
Radix Polygalae Tenuifoliae *(Yuan Zhi)*
Radix Auklandiae Lappae *(Mu Xiang)*

Er Chen Wan
Er Chen Wan means Two Aged (Ingredients) Pills. This is because two of its main ingredients are aged before use. When marketed as a dried, powdered extract, this formula is called Citrus and Pinellia Combination. This formula is used to transform phlegm and eliminate dampness. It can be added to *Xiao Yao Wan* if there is liver depression with spleen vacuity and more pronounced phlegm and dampness. If there is liver depression transforming heat giving rise to phlegm heat, it can be combined with *Dan Zhi Xiao Yao Wan.* Its ingredients are:

Rhizoma Pinelliae Ternatae *(Ban Xia)*
Sclerotium Poriae Cocos *(Fu Ling)*
Mix-fried Radix Glycyrrhizae *(Gan Cao)*
Pericarpium Citri Reticulatae *(Chen Pi)*
Uncooked Rhizoma Zingiberis *(Sheng Jiang)*

Su Zi Jiang Qi Wan
Su Zi is the name of a Chinese herb, perilla seeds. *Jiang qi* means to downbear the qi. The name of this patent medicine therefore means Perilla Seed Downbear the Qi Pills. This patent formula is usually prescribed for asthma, shortness of breath and coughs. Since it transforms phlegm and regulates the stomach qi, it can be helpful in the treatment of depression due to phlegm dampness obstruction and stagnation, especially if combined with *Xiao Yao San* in order

to treat the typically accompanying liver depression qi stagnation. Its ingredients are:

Fructus Perillae Frutescentis *(Su Zi)*
Rhizoma Pinelliae Ternatae *(Ban Xia)*
Cortex Magnoliae Officinalis *(Huo Po)*
Radix Peucedani *(Qian Hu)*
Pericarpium Citri Reticulatae *(Chen Pi)*
Lignum Aquilariae Agallochae *(Chen Xiang)*
Radix Angelicae Sinensis *(Dang Gui)*
Uncooked Rhizoma Zingiberis *(Sheng Jiang)*
Fructus Zizyphi Jujubae *(Da Zao)*
Radix Glycyrrhizae *(Gan Cao)*

Liu Wei Di Huang Wan

This formula, whose name means Six Flavours Rehmannia Pills, nourishes liver blood and kidney yin. It is the primary formula to treat symptoms of yin vacuity. It can be combined with other patent medicines in cases of depression with a strong component of yin vacuity, such as is commonly encountered around menopause or in older people. For example, these pills can be combined with *Xiao Yao Wan* or even *Dan Zhi Xiao Yao Wan*. Its ingredients are:

Cooked Radix Rehmanniae *(Shu Di)*
Fructus Corni Officinalis *(Shan Zhu Yu)*
Radix Dioscoreae Oppositae *(Shan Yao)*
Rhizoma Alismatis *(Ze Xie)*
Sclerotium Poriae Cocos *(Fu Ling)*
Cortex Radicis Moutan *(Dan Pi)*

If there are signs and symptoms of vacuity heat, then another formula should be used instead. It is made by adding the following two ingredients to the above:

Rhizoma Anemarrhenae Aspheloidis *(Zhi Mu)*
Cortex Phellodendri *(Huang Bai)*

This is then called *Zhi Bai Di Huang Wan* (Anemarrhena and Phellodendron Rehmannia Pills). For instance, *Zhi Bai Di Huang Wan* and *Bu Zhong Yi Qi Wan* (see page 85) are commonly prescribed for spleen qi vacuity, liver depression, kidney yin vacuity and yin vacuity and/or damp heat, i.e. the complex yin fire scenario we talked about above.

Jin Gui Shen Qi Wan

The name of these commonly available Chinese patent pills translates as Golden Cabinet Kidney Qi Pills. The 'golden cabinet' is an allusion to the name of the book this formula is first recorded in, *Jin Gui Yao Lue (Essentials from the Golden Cabinet),* dating from 200–250 AD. This is the most well-known formula for the treatment of kidney yang vacuity and it can be combined with other formulae when kidney yang vacuity complicates a patient's pattern discrimination. Its ingredients include:

Cooked Radix Rehmanniae *(Shu Di)*
Fructus Corni Officinalis *(Shan Zhu Yu)*
Radix Dioscoreae Oppositae *(Shan Yao)*
Sclerotium Poriae Cocos *(Fu Ling)*
Rhizoma Alismatis *(Ze Xie)*
Cortex Radicis Moutan *(Dan Pi)*
Radix Lateralis Praeparatus Aconiti Carmichaeli *(Fu Zi)*
Cortex Cinnamomi Cassiae *(Rou Gui)*

This formula contains prepared Chinese aconite *(Fu Zi),* which is one of the most fundamental and important herbs used in Chinese medicine. Unfortunately it may not be available in the UK as the current legislative guidelines do not allow the internal use of a related species of European aconite in an unprepared form. Whilst Chinese herbalists hope that this situation will be remedied in the future, for the moment this well-known and vital formula may not be used in the UK. It should be said that prepared aconite is a dynamic and powerful herb and should never be used without professional diagnosis and advice. Both prepared aconite and cinnamon *(Rou Gui)* are warming or hot herbs, which is why they are so effective in raising the yang energy of the body. This formula may be particularly helpful for the elderly whose yang energy has decreased. It has a good balance of herbs to nourish the yin, too.

Tian Wang Bu Xin Dan

The name of this formula translates as Heavenly Emperor's Supplement the Heart Elixir. This formula comes as a Chinese patent medicine in pill form. When marketed as a desiccated, powdered extract, this formula is sold under the name Ginseng and Zizyphus Formula. It treats insomnia, restlessness, fatigue and heart palpitations due to yin, blood and qi vacuity, with an emphasis on heart yin and liver blood vacuity. Its ingredients include:

Uncooked Radix Rehmanniae *(Sheng Di)*
Radix Scrophulariae Ningpoensis *(Xuan Shen)*
Fructus Schisandrae Chinensis *(Wu Wei Zi)*
Tuber Asparagi Cochinensis *(Tian Men Dong)*
Tuber Ophiopogonis Japonici *(Mai Men Dong)*
Radix Angelicae Sinensis *(Dang Gui)*
Semen Biotae Orientalis *(Bai Zi Ren)*
Semen Zizyphi Spinosae *(Suan Zao Ren)*
Radix Salviae Miltiorrhizae *(Dan Shen)*
Radix Polygalae Tenuifoliae *(Yuan Zhi)*
Sclerotium Poriae Cocos *(Fu Ling)*
Radix Codonopsitis Pilosulae *(Dang Shen)*

***Bai Zi Yang Xin Wan* (also spelt *Pai Tsu Yang Hsin Wan*)**

The name of this formula translates as Biota Seed Nourish the Heart Pills. This is another commonly used over-the-counter Chinese patent pill. It is usually marketed for insomnia, but it can be helpful when depression is characterised by heart yin and liver blood vacuity complicated by an element of phlegm obstruction. If liver depression qi stagnation or liver depression transforming heat complicate the scenario, this formula can be combined with *Xiao Yao Wan* or *Dan Zhi Xiao Yao Wan* respectively. Its ingredients include:

Semen Biotae Orientalis *(Bai Zi Ren)*
Fructus Lycii Chinensis *(Gou Qi Zi)*
Radix Scrophulariae Ningpoensis *(Xuan Shen)*
Uncooked Radix Rehmanniae *(Sheng Di)*
Tuber Ophiopogonis Japonici *(Mai Men Dong)*
Radix Angelicae Sinensis *(Dang Gui)*
Sclerotium Poriae Cocos *(Fu Ling)*
Rhizoma Acori Graminei *(Shi Chang Pu)*
Radix Glycyrrhizae *(Gan Cao)*

Tabellae *Suan Zao Ren Tang*
This is the tablet or pill form of a famous spirit-calming Chinese medicinal decoction, Zizyphus Spinosa Decoction. Its ingredients are:

Semen Zizyphi Spinosae *(Suan Zao Ren)*
Radix Ligustici Wallichii *(Chuan Xiong)*
Sclerotium Poriae Cocos *(Fu Ling)*
Rhizoma Anemarrhenae Aspheloidis *(Zhi Mu)*
Radix Glycyrrhizae *(Gan Cao)*

This formula is for insomnia and restlessness or anxiety due primarily to liver blood vacuity with possibly a little heat disturbing the heart spirit. It can be added to any of the liver depression formulae suggested above.

Ding Xin Wan
The name of this Chinese patent pill translates as Stabilise the Heart Pills. It supplements the heart qi and blood, quiets the heart spirit and clears heat disturbing the heart from the liver and/or stomach. It can be taken in combination with liver depression and transformative heat formulae described

above where heart qi and blood vacuity with transformative heat leads to restless spirit, anxiety, heart palpitations and insomnia. Its ingredients include:

Radix Codonopsitis Pilosulae *(Dang Shen)*
Radix Angelicae Sinensis *(Dang Gui)*
Sclerotium Pararadicis Poriae Cocos *(Fu Shen)*
Radix Polygalae Tenuifoliae *(Yuan Zhi)*
Semen Zizyphi Spinosae *(Suan Zao Ren)*
Semen Biotae Orientalis *(Bai Zi Ren)*
Radix Scutellariae Baicalensis *(Huang Qin)*
Tuber Ophiopogonis Japonici *(Mai Men Dong)*
Succinum *(Hu Po)*

An Mian Pian
These are called Quiet Sleep Pills. They can be used by themselves or combined with other appropriate patent pills for insomnia and restlessness due to liver depression transforming heat and liver blood not nourishing the heart spirit. Their ingredients are:

Semen Zizyphi Spinosae *(Suan Zao Ren)*
Radix Polygalae Tenuifoliae *(Yuan Zhi)*
Sclerotium Poriae Cocos *(Fu Ling)*
Fructus Gardeniae Jasminoidis *(Shan Zhi Zi)*
Massa Medica Fermentata *(Shen Qu)*
Radix Glycyrrhizae *(Gan Cao)*

***Tong Jing Wan* (also spelt *To Jing Wan*)**
The name of these pills means Painful Menstruation Pills. Depression is often complicated by blood stasis in women and the elderly. The symptoms of blood stasis include painful menstruation with the passage of dark clots, pain that is stabbing or intense in nature and tends to be fixed in position, a dark, dusky facial complexion, possible black circles under the eyes, purplish lips, a purplish tongue, possible static blood patches or dots on the tongue, broken blood vessels, small,

red nodules on the skin, varicosities, inflammation of veins, piles and a bowstring, choppy pulse. In such cases, this pill can be taken along with other appropriate formulae when blood stasis is an important factor in someone's depression. Its ingredients are:

Tuber Curcumae *(Yu Jin)*
Rhizoma Sparganii *(San Leng)*
Radix Rubrus Paeoniae Lactiflorae *(Chi Shao)*
Radix Angelicae Sinensis *(Dang Gui)*
Radix Ligustici Wallichii *(Chuan Xiong)*
Radix Salviae Miltiorrhizae *(Dan Shen)*
Flos Carthami Tinctorii *(Hong Hua)*

Xue Fu Zhu Yu Wan

The name of these pills means Blood Mansion Dispels Stasis Pills. They are yet another Chinese patent medicine in pill form for the treatment of blood stasis. This formula is the one that Wu and Bai suggest for liver blood stasis and stagnation emotional depression. Its ingredients include:

Semen Pruni Persicae *(Tao Ren)*
Radix Angelicae Sinensis *(Dang Gui)*
Flos Carthami Tinctorii *(Hong Hua)*
Uncooked Radix Rehmanniae *(Sheng Di)*
Radix Achyranthis Bidentatae *(Niu Xi)*
Radix Ligustici Wallichii *(Chuan Xiong)*
Radix Rubrus Paeoniae Lactiflorae *(Chi Shao)*
Fructus Citri Aurantii *(Zhi Ke)*
Radix Bupleuri *(Chai Hu)*
Radix Platycodi Grandiflori *(Jie Geng)*
Radix Glycyrrhizae *(Gan Cao)*

Bu Zhong Yi Qi Wan

The name of this formula translates as Supplement the Centre and Boost the Qi Decoction. It strongly supplements spleen vacuity. It is commonly used to treat central qi fall, i.e.

prolapse of the stomach, uterus or rectum due to spleen qi vacuity. It is a very complex formula with a wide range of indications. It supplements the spleen but also courses the liver and rectifies the qi. It is very commonly prescribed and these pills can be combined with a number of others when spleen qi vacuity and liver depression play a significant role in someone's depression (without signs of significant blood vacuity or more severe dampness). Its ingredients are:

Radix Astragali Membranacei *(Huang Qi)*
Radix Panacis Ginseng *(Ren Shen)*
Radix Glycyrrhizae *(Gan Cao)*
Rhizoma Atractylodis Macrocephalae *(Bai Zhu)*
Radix Angelicae Sinensis *(Dang Gui)*
Pericarpium Citri Reticulatae *(Chen Pi)*
Rhizoma Cimicifugae *(Sheng Ma)*
Radix Bupleuri *(Chai Hu)*
Rhizoma Atractylodis Macrocephalae *(Bai Zhu)*

All the formulae mentioned so far are commonly used and well known for their ability to treat different patterns of depression. Availability depends on the legislation governing herbal medicine in the country in which you live. In the USA, they are available over the counter at health food stores and at Asian speciality food stores. In Europe, legislation is different and the herbs may not be available without a prescription from a qualified practitioner of Chinese medicine. As mentioned previously, Chinese herbal medicines can be powerful and dynamic. They have the power to heal and therefore the potential to harm if incorrectly used.

ASSESSING OVER-THE-COUNTER MEDICATION

If you do try Chinese herbal patent medicines for your depression without professional guidance, please be careful.

Be sure to follow these guidelines for assessing the safety of any medications you take.

In general, you can tell if any medication and treatment is appropriate for you by checking the following six aspects of your health:

Digestion
Elimination
Energy level
Mood
Appetite
Sleep

If a medication, be it modern Western or traditional Chinese, alleviates your symptoms and these six basic areas of health also improve, then it is probably a good treatment. However, if a treatment or medication causes a deterioration in any of these six mechanisms, even if there is an improvement in your symptoms, then it is probably not the correct treatment and certainly should not be taken on a long-term basis. Chinese medicine aims to rebalance the body's energies and create harmony allowing the body's own natural healing mechanisms to be reinstated. Nothing is more powerful than nature's own healing, and this is healing without side-effects.

ACUPUNCTURE AND ORIENTAL MEDICAL MASSAGE

In the previous chapters we have looked at the underlying causes of depression from a traditional Chinese medicine (TCM) point of view and its treatment with internal or herbal medicine. This chapter will focus on how Chinese medicine treats depression using acupuncture and Oriental medical massage. Chinese medicine as it has evolved in China has developed in a different social and cultural context from the West and there are differences in how it is practised. In modern China, herbal treatment is very popular. In fact, TCM has evolved principally from a herbal tradition. In the West there have been many other influences, and whilst TCM has played an important role other countries such as Japan have also been influential. Shiatsu, for example, a type of Oriental medical massage originating from Japan, is very popular in the West today and can be a very helpful therapy for depression. Acupuncture is probably the most well-known and widely practised form of medicine in the UK, having been practised since the 1960s. It has grown enormously in popularity and there are now many trained practitioners all over the country. We will look at how to find a properly qualified practitioner later on in the book.

WHAT IS ACUPUNCTURE?

Acupuncture involves the insertion of extremely fine needles into specific points on the body along channels or pathways that correspond to the yin viscera and yang bowels we mentioned earlier. By stimulating these points an acupuncturist may influence the flow of qi, or energy, in the pathway thereby influencing the function of the corresponding viscus or bowel. Since all the viscera and bowels work together as a team, this then influences the whole energetic system of the person. The aim of acupuncture is to regulate the flow of qi so that there is more balance and harmony in the pathways or channels. Acupuncture can be very beneficial for treating depression because it improves the flow of qi. As discussed earlier, this can be important in depression, particularly if there is liver depression qi stagnation involved, as is often the case. Acupuncture may help to rectify and balance the flow of qi in the body and thereby improve overall health as well as relieve or improve specific symptoms

As a generic term, acupuncture also includes several other methods (apart from the use of needles) for stimulating acupuncture points, thus regulating the flow of qi in the body. One of the other main methods is moxibustion (see page 119). This means the warming of acupuncture points mainly by burning dried, aged Oriental mugwort on, near or over acupuncture points. The purpose of this warming treatment is to stimulate the flow of qi and blood even more strongly, to add warmth to areas of the body which are too cold and to add yang qi to the body to supplement a yang qi deficiency. Some other methods or techniques to stimulate the points that may be used by the acupuncturist are cupping, electro-acupuncture and the application of magnets.

What is a typical acupuncture treatment for depression like?

There are quite a few styles of acupuncture so some aspects of treatment will vary from practitioner to practitioner depending on their training, but there are also certain aspects that remain the same. All practitioners will take a case history and gather together information so that they can make a diagnosis. They will almost certainly take the pulse at the wrist, examine the tongue and palpate the abdomen and the 'channels', looking for areas of tenderness or pain. Once a diagnosis has been made, the practitioner will select points along the channels and will stimulate these points with needles, moxa and possibly some of the other stimulation methods mentioned earlier. These days most acupuncturists use disposable needles and all members of the professional bodies listed in this book must comply with strict standards of hygiene and safety. An acupuncture needle is extremely fine, nothing like a hypodermic needle, and although pain thresholds vary from person to person it is not necessarily a painful therapy. The effect of the treatment may be quite relaxing or even stimulating as the qi is able to flow more freely in the body.

In China, acupuncture treatments are given every day or every other day, three to five times a week, depending on the nature and severity of the condition. In the West, most people visit their practitioner once or twice a week at first and then attend less frequently as their health improves. After an acute episode of depression has passed, patients are strongly advised to maintain acupuncture treatment once a month in order to prevent any relapses, as depression tends to be a recurrent condition. In general, improvements are gradual and progressive, because the therapy is working by enhancing the person's own natural healing mechanisms rather than by symptom relief. We have found in our clinical experience that when acupuncture is combined with appropriate lifestyle changes and possibly herbal medication, the progress can be more rapid.

How are the points selected?

The points where the acupuncturist chooses to manipulate a needle during treatment are selected on the basis of Chinese medical theory and the known clinical effects of certain points. As mentioned earlier, there are different styles of practice, and point selection may vary from practitioner to practitioner. In order to illustrate how an acupuncture treatment works, we will use the case of Joan and show how a practitioner working with TCM might select the points according to the pattern discrimination. TCM is probably one of the main methods of practising acupuncture, and is widely used in the USA and the UK. However, it is not the only one, so don't worry if your practitioner is not trained in this method or chooses to work in a different way. Diversity of practice is very important in Oriental medicine and enriches the whole field.

Case history

In Joan's case her main complaints were irritability, increased appetite and weight gain, lethargy, apathy and difficulty sleeping. We have previously established that Joan's pattern discrimination according to TCM was one of liver depression transforming into heat which is then harassing the stomach and heart, complicated by dampness and phlegm due to spleen qi vacuity.

The appropriate treatment principles to help in Joan's case are to course the liver, rectify and boost the qi, clear heat, fortify the spleen, eliminate dampness, transform phlegm and 'calm' her spirit. In order to accomplish these aims, the practitioner might select the following points:

Tai Chong (Liver 3)
He Gu (Large Intestine 4)
San Yin Jiao (Spleen 6)
Shen Men (Heart 7)
Nei Guan (Pericardium 6)
Jiu Wei (Conception Vessel 15)
Feng Long (Stomach 40)
Shen Ting (Governing Vessel 24)
Ben Shen (Gall bladder 20)

The actions of these selected points are as follows:

Tai Chong courses the liver, resolves depression and moves and rectifies the qi. Since liver depression qi stagnation is fundamental to Joan's depression, this is a vital point in this treatment. It will have a calming effect and soothe Joan's irritability and anger.

He Gu is a widely used point with a variety of indications depending on how it is used and with what points it is combined. When combined with *Tai Chong*, the treatment is known as 'the four gates'. This is a powerful treatment used to enhance and free the flow of qi throughout the entire body. *He Gu* is also chosen as it has the ability to clear heat from the upper part of the body and to promote the 'bearing up of the clear' and 'bearing down of the turbid' by the qi mechanism. This means it is able to regulate the elimination of waste (it is on the large intestine channel).

San Yin Jiao is chosen as it benefits both the liver and the spleen. Both these channels cross at this point on the lower leg.

Shen Men is a point on the heart channel that benefits the heart. It clears heat from the heart and calms the heart spirit.

Nei Guan is a point on the pericardium channel. The pericardium performs many vital functions within the body–mind–spirit. It is sometimes translated as the 'heart protector' and does work closely with the heart and circulation. This point is selected because it frees the flow of qi in the chest and calms or quiets the spirit in the heart. These two points, *Shen Men* and *Nei Guan*, are frequently used for the treatment of various patterns of depression.

Jiu Wei is a point on the front centre line of the body located just under the diaphragm. It is very helpful in alleviating depression, particularly if there are symptoms of chest oppression. It is also very helpful in calming the spirit.

Feng Long is a point on the stomach channel. The stomach and spleen work very closely together according to Chinese medicine, and this point will benefit both as it is said to connect them to each other. The stomach channel travels over the chest so this will help with the flow of qi in this area. It can also support the spleen and help to transform phlegm and dampness.

Shen Ting is selected as it helps quiet the spirit, open the orifices and arouse the brain, while *Ben Shen* is a point on the gall bladder channel that courses the liver and lifts depression. Using both these points together is a very effective combination for treating depression when liver qi stagnation is involved.

These nine points have been selected as they will benefit Joan according to her Chinese medical pattern diagnosis. Other points could also be chosen should certain symptoms predominate over the course of her treatment, so she will not necessarily receive the same treatment on each occasion. The treatment will aim to improve Joan's symptoms as well as working to benefit her overall health and well-being.

Who should receive acupuncture?

Acupuncture will probably benefit anyone who suffers from depression. Its effect on moving the stuck (blocked) qi often brings immediate relief. If someone is very depleted in their energy and has more signs of severe qi, blood or yin vacuity or depletion, then acupuncture alone may not be enough to help. The best that treatment with acupuncture can achieve is to stimulate and support the viscera and bowels that create and transform the qi, blood and yin. Treatment with Chinese herbs, however, actually puts something substantial into the body and can directly supplement deficiencies of the qi, blood and yin. Treatment with acupuncture is basically very helpful and supportive for depression but may not be sufficient in some cases. Your practitioner will be able to advise you best, bearing in mind your individual circumstances.

EAR ACUPUNCTURE

Some acupuncturists may also use points in the ear to treat depression. Needles may be used during the acupuncture session or alternatively tiny metal pellets, seeds or special 'press tac' needles are used, which are covered up with tape and left in place for a few days. In this way the effectiveness and duration of treatment may be enhanced.

In terms of depression, the point on the ear known as *Shen Men*[6] can have a profound effect by relaxing tension and irritability and also improving sleep. There are also other points, such as the Sympathetic Point, the Brain Point and the Subcortex Point that can be very helpful in the treatment of depression.

ORIENTAL MEDICAL MASSAGE

Medical massage in China is called *tui na.* It has developed into a high art and is practised extensively in hospitals and clinics. Like acupuncture it works by stimulating the flow of qi in the channel or meridian system except instead of needles, specific strokes or manipulations are used. At present there are not many trained *tui na* practitioners in the UK although it is growing in popularity. Another form of Oriental medical massage is shiatsu, which originates from Japan. This is a deeply relaxing therapy and there are a number of practitioners working in the UK. Shiatsu is performed with the patient wearing loose, comfortable clothing. Diagnosis is mainly through palpating the abdomen and channels to detect underlying imbalances in the person's energy. The relevant channels or meridians are then worked on to release blockages and strengthen areas of vacuity or deficiency. It may be very beneficial for depression. Oriental medical massage can stimulate the flow of qi and also make someone feel better about themselves. Being touched can in itself be very healing.

---

[6] This point shares the same name as Heart 7 but is located on the ear. The English translation of *Shen Men* is 'Spirit Gate'.

THE THREE FREE THERAPIES

All the treatments and therapies we have so far discussed require the aid of a professional practitioner. There are, however, three 'free therapies' that are crucial to treating depression. These are diet, exercise and deep relaxation. Only you can take care of these three factors in your health!

DIET

In Chinese medicine, the functions of the spleen and stomach are likened to a pot on a stove or a tank in a still. The stomach receives the foods and liquids which then 'rot and ripen' like a mash in a fermentation vat. The spleen then cooks this mash and drives off (i.e. transforms and moves upwards) the pure part. This pure part collects in the lungs to become the qi and in the heart to become the blood. Chinese medicine characterises this transformation as a process of yang qi transforming yin substance. All the principles of Chinese dietary therapy that may be applied to treat and alleviate depression are derived from these basic theories.

We have already seen that the spleen is fundamental to the creation of qi and blood. Based on this concept, a healthy, strong spleen prevents and treats depression in four ways. First of all, fatigue is always a symptom of qi vacuity. Second, if the spleen is healthy and strong, it will create sufficient qi to push the blood and move body fluids. A sufficient amount of pushing or moving spleen qi helps counterbalance or control any tendency of the liver to constrict or constrain the qi flow. This means that a healthy spleen helps keep the liver in check and free from depression and stagnation. Third, since the spleen is the root of blood production and it is yin blood that keeps yang qi in check, a healthy, strong spleen manufacturing abundant blood ensures a sufficient amount of 'heart' blood to nourish and quiet the spirit. And fourth, since all qi and especially blood remaining unused at the end of the day can be converted into essence during sleep at night, a strong, healthy spleen, which manufactures abundant qi and blood, helps ensure the supplementation of yin by this acquired essence.

With regard to Chinese dietary therapy and depression, the fundamental principle is to avoid foods that damage the spleen. These foods also typically produce dampness and phlegm.

Foods that damage the spleen

In terms of foods that damage the spleen we begin with uncooked and especially chilled foods. In Chinese medicine the process of digestion is likened to cooking, which is seen as a type of predigestion before the food enters the body. It is therefore desirable that the overwhelming majority of all food should be cooked, i.e. predigested. Although cooking may destroy some vital nutrients (or qi), cooking does render the remaining nutrients more easily assimilated. This means that even though some nutrients have been lost, the net absorption of nutrients is greater with cooked foods than raw. Furthermore, eating raw foods makes the spleen work harder and can overtax it. If your spleen is very robust, eating uncooked, raw foods may not be too damaging. However, women in particular need to take extra care as their monthly menses and resulting extra blood production may already be overtaxing the spleen. It is also a fact of life according to Chinese medicine that the spleen typically weakens with age.

Chilled foods even more than raw foods may directly damage the spleen. Chilled or frozen foods and drinks neutralise the spleen's yang qi. The process of digestion involves warming and transforming all food and drink to a 100°F soup within the stomach so that it may undergo 'distillation'. If the spleen expends too much yang qi just warming the food up, then it will become damaged and weak. So food and drink should be consumed at room temperature at the least and preferably at body temperature. The more signs and symptoms of spleen vacuity or deficiency that a person presents, such as fatigue, chronically loose stools, undigested food in the stools, cold hands and feet, dizziness on standing up and aversion to cold, the more they need to avoid uncooked, chilled food and drink.

Additionally, an excess of sugars and sweet things directly damages the spleen. It is considered that they are inherently dampening according to Chinese medicine. This is because the body creates or secretes fluids that collect, transforming into dampness, in response to an excess of sweet food and drink. The spleen is averse to dampness. Dampness is a yin substance and controls or checks yang qi, which is very important to the proper functioning of the spleen. So anything that is excessively dampening damages the spleen. The sweeter a food is, the more dampening and therefore more damaging it is to the spleen.

There are two other food categories that are considered to be dampening and subsequently damage the spleen.

'Sodden wheat foods': this means flour products such as bread and noodles. Wheat (as opposed to rice) is damp in its nature. When it is steamed, yeasted and/or refined, it becomes even more damp.

Oils and fats: the more oily or greasy a food is, the worse it is for the spleen. As milk contains a lot of fat, dairy products fall into this category. This includes milk, butter and cheese.

If we add all this up, then ice cream is just about the worst thing a person with a weak, damp spleen could eat. Ice cream is chilled, it is intensely sweet and it is filled with fat. So it is a triple whammy when it comes to damaging the spleen. In the same way, pasta smothered in tomato sauce and cheese is a recipe for disaster. Pasta made from wheat flour is dampening, tomatoes are dampening and cheese is dampening. Most people don't realise that a glass of fruit juice contains as much sugar as a sweet bar, so fruit juice is also very damaging to the spleen and produces damp.

As we have seen, most cases of depression involve an element of liver depression and qi stagnation. Stagnant qi leads to stagnation of other substances, such as dampness and phlegm. It is not unusual to encounter a pattern of depression that involves both a loss of the liver's ability to course and discharge (resulting in a stagnation of qi) and a weakening of the spleen's ability to transport and transform (which results in dampness and phlegm). In our clinical experience, a great number of people who experience depression react very favourably to the elimination of both wheat and dairy products from their diet and, in some cases, to the elimination of other gluten-rich grains, such as oats and barley.

Below is a list of specific Western foods that are either uncooked, chilled, too sweet or too dampening and thus damaging to the spleen. People with depression should minimise their consumption of these or avoid them, especially if they know their spleen is weak.

Ice cream
Sugar
Sweets, especially chocolate
Milk
Butter
Cheese
Margarine
Yoghurt
Raw salads
Fruit juices
Juicy, sweet fruits, such as oranges, peaches, strawberries and tomatoes
Fatty meats
Fried foods
Refined flour products
Cakes and biscuits

Yeasted bread
Nuts
Alcohol (which is essentially sugar)

If the spleen is weak and wet, it is best not to eat too much of anything at any one time. A weak spleen can be overwhelmed by a large meal, especially if any of the food is hard to digest. This then results in food stagnation which impedes the free flow of qi all the more and causes further damage to the spleen.

A clear, bland diet

In Chinese medicine, the best diet for the spleen and, by extension, the best diet for most people, is what is called a 'clear, bland diet'. This is a diet high in complex carbohydrates such as unrefined grains, especially rice and beans. It is high in lightly cooked vegetables. It is a diet that is low in fatty meats, oily, greasy, fried foods and very sweet foods. It is not, however, a completely vegetarian diet. Most people, in our experience, should eat one to two ounces of various types of meat two to four times per week. This animal flesh could be chicken and fish, but should also include some lean beef, pork and lamb. Some fresh or cooked fruits may be eaten, but fruit juices should be avoided. Women especially should make an effort to include tofu and tempeh in their diet, two soya foods now commonly available in health food shops and good supermarkets.

If the spleen is weak, then it is best to eat smaller, more frequent meals. Rice is also an excellent food, for three reasons: it is neutral in temperature, it fortifies the spleen thereby supplementing the qi and it eliminates dampness. Rice should be the main or staple grain in the diet.

A few problem foods

There are a few 'problem' foods which deserve special mention.

Coffee

The first of these is coffee. Many people crave coffee for two reasons. Firstly, coffee moves stuck qi. So, if a person suffers from liver depression qi stagnation, coffee will temporarily make them feel as if their qi is flowing. Secondly, coffee transforms essence into qi and makes that qi temporarily available to the body. This means that people who suffer from spleen and/or kidney vacuity fatigue will get a temporary lift from coffee. It will make them feel as if they have energy. Once this energy is used up, they are left with a deficit. The coffee has transformed some of the essence stored in the kidneys into qi. This qi has been used and now there is less stored essence. Since the blood and essence share a common source, coffee drinking may ultimately worsen depression associated with blood or kidney vacuities. Tea has a similar effect in that it transforms yin essence into yang qi but the quantity of caffeine in tea is usually only half that found in coffee.

Chocolate

Chocolate is a combination of oil, sugar and cocoa. We have seen that both oil and sugar are dampening and damaging to the spleen. Temporarily, the sugar will boost the spleen qi, but ultimately it will result in 'sugar blues' or a hypoglycaemic letdown. Cocoa stirs the life gate fire, another name for kidney yang or kidney fire, and kidney fire is the source of sexual energy and desire. It is said that chocolate is the food of love and, from the Chinese medical point of view, that is true. Since chocolate stimulates kidney fire at the same time as it temporarily boosts the spleen, it does give one a rush of yang qi. This rush of yang qi does move depression and stagnation, at least in the short term. So it makes sense that some people with liver depression, spleen vacuity and kidney yang debility might crave chocolate.

Alcohol

Alcohol is both damp and hot according to Chinese medical theory. It strongly moves the qi and blood. So people with liver depression qi stagnation will feel temporarily better after drinking alcohol. However, the sugar in alcohol damages the spleen and creates dampness, which 'gums up the works', whilst the heat (yang) in alcohol can waste the blood (yin) and aggravate or inflame depressive liver heat.

Hot, peppery foods

Spicy, peppery foods also move the qi, thereby giving some temporary relief to liver depression qi stagnation. However, like alcohol, the heat in spicy, hot foods wastes the blood and can inflame yang.

Sour foods

In Chinese medicine, the sour flavour is inherently astringent and constricting. People with liver depression qi stagnation should be careful not to use vinegar and other intensely sour foods, which will only aggravate the qi stagnation by astringent and further restricting the qi and blood. This is also why sweet and sour foods, such as orange juice and tomatoes, are particularly bad for people with liver depression and spleen vacuity. The sour flavour constricts the qi, while the sweet flavour damages the spleen and creates dampness.

Diet drinks

Diet drinks containing artificial sweeteners seem to contain something that damages the Chinese concept of the kidneys. A number of patients over the years have reported that, when they drink a lot of diet drinks they experience urinary incontinence and lower back and knee pain and weakness. If they stop, these symptoms disappear. Taken as a group, according to Chinese medicine, these are kidney vacuity symptoms. Since many people aged 40 and above suffering from depression have concomitant kidney vacuity, they are recommended to steer clear of diet drinks so as not to weaken the kidneys any further or faster.

Foods that help nourish the blood

Qi and Wei

According to Chinese dietary therapy, all foods contain both qi and wei in varying amounts. Qi means the ability to catalyse or promote yang function, while wei (literally translated as flavour) refers to a food's ability to nourish or construct yin substance. Since blood is relatively yin compared to qi being yang, a certain amount of food high in wei is necessary for a person to create and transform blood. Foods that are high in wei as compared to qi are those that tend to be heavy, dense, greasy or oily, meaty or bloody. All animal products contain more wei than vegetable products. Black beans and, even better, black soya beans contain more wei than, say, celery or lettuce.

When people suffer from depression and anxiety because of blood vacuity failing to nourish the heart and quiet the spirit, or yin vacuity failing to control yang, they usually need to eat slightly more foods high in wei. This includes animal proteins and products, such as meat and eggs. It is said that flesh foods are very 'compassionate' to the human body. This word recognises the fact that the animal's life has had to be sacrificed to produce this type of food. It also recognises that, because such food is so close to the human body itself, it is especially nutritious. Eating some animal products can therefore be helpful and might even be necessary when people suffer from depression with blood and yin vacuity.

Animal foods versus vegetarianism

Based on many years of clinical experience, Bob Flaws has observed many Westerners who adhere to a strict vegetarian diet and who after several years develop blood or yin vacuity patterns. This is especially the case in women who lose blood every month and must build babies out of the blood and yin essence. When women who are strict vegetarians present with the signs and symptoms of blood vacuity, such as a thick, pale tongue, pale face, pale nails and pale lips, heart palpitations, insomnia and fatigue with a fine, forceless pulse, it is recommended that they include a little animal food in their diet. They often report how much better they feel once they have made these dietary changes, and notice that they have much more energy.

The downside of eating meat, apart from ethical issues, is that foods that are high in wei also tend to be harder to digest and to create phlegm and dampness. It is best that such foods only be eaten in very small amounts at any one time. The weaker the person's spleen or the more phlegm and dampness they already have, the less of such foods they should eat.

Remember we said above that the process of digestion first consisted of turning the food and drink ingested into a 100°F soup in the stomach. Soups and broths made out of animal flesh are the easiest and most digestible way of adding some animal-quality wei to the diet. When eating flesh itself, this should probably be limited to only one to two ounces per serving and only three or four such servings per week. According to Chinese dietary principles, the best meats for creating and transforming blood and yin essence are organ meats and red or dark meats. This includes beef, venison and lamb, and dark meat from chicken, turkey, goose and duck. White pork meat is also fine, as is ham. White fish and white meat from poultry are less effective for building blood.

One good recipe for adding more digestible wei to the diet of a person who is blood vacuous is to take a marrow bone and boil this with some cut vegetables, especially root vegetables, and black beans or black soya beans. Such a soup is easy to digest and yet rich in wei.

The proverbial glass of hot milk

The fact that milk is rich in wei is exactly why it induces sleep or is soporific according to Chinese medicine. Being high in wei or yin, milk helps control counterflowing, hyperactive yang. The Chinese would say that blending a whole egg into boiling milk makes this time-tested remedy even more effective for enriching yin. In depression cases where liver depression qi stagnation combines with significant yin vacuity, and insomnia is one of the main symptoms, drinking some warm milk before bedtime may actually help the insomnia as long as the person does not suffer from either dampness or phlegm. For people with phlegm heat pattern depression that also presents with insomnia, drinking a warm glass of milk before bed will typically make both their depression and their insomnia worse! This is the beauty of Chinese medicine. It allows one to determine on an individual basis whether any food, medicine or activity will be appropriate for a particular pattern of imbalance.

The most important thing to remember about diet is that if the spleen is healthy and strong, then you will manufacture good amounts of qi and blood as long as you eat primarily a clear, bland diet with a little bit of animal food, and take sufficient exercise without overexerting yourself. Whatever of this qi and blood is left unconsumed at the end of the day will be transformed into acquired essence that night. This is the safest way of producing and transforming blood and yin – via the diet. If you consume an excess of foods that are high in wei, in theory these may supplement yin and nourish blood but they will also gum up the qi mechanism. The net result will be less qi and blood, not more, and the situation will be further complicated by the creation of more phlegm and dampness.

In the following chapter, there are some specific recipes combining Chinese herbs and foods for regulating the qi and quieting the spirit to help depression.

Some last words on diet

In conclusion, Western patients are always asking what they should eat in order to cure their disease. Unfortunately, when it comes to diet, the issue is not so much what to eat as what not to eat. Diet most definitely plays a major role in the cause and perpetuation of many people's depression, but, except in the case of vegetarians suffering from blood or yin vacuities, the issue is mainly what to avoid or minimise, not what to add. Most of us know that coffee, chocolate, sugars, sweets, oils, fats and alcohol are not good for us. Most of us know that we should be eating more complex carbohydrates and freshly cooked vegetables and less fatty meats. However, it's one thing to know these things and another to follow what we know.

To be perfectly honest, a clear, bland diet as recommended according to the principles of Chinese medicine is not the most exciting diet in the world. It is, however, quite a traditional type of diet and many of our great-grandparents would have eaten like this. Our modern Western diet, which is high in oils and fats, high in sugars and sweets, high in animal proteins and proportionally high in uncooked, chilled foods and drinks, is a relatively recent phenomenon and you can't fool Mother Nature.

When you change to the clear, bland diet of Chinese medicine, you might find that at first you suffer from cravings for more tasty food. These cravings are, in many cases, actually associated with food 'allergies'. We may crave what is actually not good for us in the same way that an alcoholic craves for alcohol. After a few days, these cravings tend to disappear and you can find that you don't miss some of the convenience or 'comfort' foods as much as you thought you would. Perseverance is the key to long-term success. As the Chinese say, 'A million is made up of nothing but lots of ones and a bucket is quickly filled by steady drips and drops.'

EXERCISE

Exercise is the second of the three 'free' therapies. According to Chinese medicine, regular and adequate exercise has two basic benefits. Firstly, exercise promotes the movement of the qi and quickening of the blood. Since almost all depression involves liver depression qi stagnation, it is obvious that exercise is an important therapy for coursing the liver and rectifying the qi. Secondly, exercise benefits the spleen. The spleen's movement and transportation of digested food is dependent upon the qi mechanism. The qi mechanism describes the function of the qi in moving up and down the pure and turbid parts of digestion respectively. For the qi mechanism to function properly, the qi must be flowing normally and freely. Since exercise moves and rectifies the qi, it also helps regulate and rectify the qi mechanism. The result is that the spleen is able to function well, creating and transforming qi and blood. Spleen qi vacuity and dampness accumulation typically complicates depression; a healthy spleen is able to control a 'depressed' liver. Regular, adequate exercise is vitally important for either preventing or treating depression.

Aerobics

In our experience, aerobic exercise is found to be the most beneficial for the majority of people with depression. By aerobic exercise, we mean any physical activity that raises the heartbeat 80 per cent above normal resting rate and keeps it there for at least 20 minutes. To calculate your normal resting heart rate, place your fingers over the pulsing artery on the front side of your neck. Count the beats for 15 seconds and then multiply by four. This gives you your beats per minute or BPM. Now multiply your BPM by 0.8. Take the resulting number and add it to your resting BPM. This gives you your aerobic threshold of BPM. Next engage in any physical activity you like. After you have been exercising for five minutes, take your pulse for 15 seconds once again at the artery on the front side of your throat. Again multiply the resulting count by four to find your current BPM. If this number is less than your aerobic threshold BPM, then you know you need to exercise harder or faster. Once you get your heart rate up to your aerobic threshold, then you need to keep exercising at the same level of intensity for at least 20 minutes. Take your pulse every five minutes or so to ensure your heartbeat is being kept high enough.

Depending on your age and physical condition, you will require different types of exercise to reach your aerobic threshold. For some, simply walking briskly will raise the heartbeat 80 per cent above its resting rate. Others will need to do callisthenics, running, swimming, squash or some other, more strenuous exercise. It really does not matter what the exercise is as long as it raises your heartbeat 80 per cent above your resting rate and keeps it there for 20 minutes. My advice is that you go for something you enjoy and don't find too boring otherwise you won't want to keep it up. You should also try to make sure that it doesn't cause you any problems or damage to any parts of the body. For example, running on pavements may cause knee problems for some people.

When doing aerobic exercise, it is best to exercise either every day or every other day. If you do not do your aerobics at least once every 72 hours, then its cumulative effects won't be as good. I recommend that my patients with depression do some sort of aerobic exercises every day or every other day, three to four times per week at least. The good news is that there is no real need to exercise more than 30 minutes at any one time. A session of 45 minutes is not going to be all that much better than 25 minutes, and 25 minutes four times a week is very much better than one hour once a week.

Weight-lifting

Recent research has also demonstrated that weight-lifting can help relieve depression in women of all ages. It might be beneficial to try and schedule some weight-lifting into your exercise routine. I suggest that you do aerobics three to four days a week and lift weights on the other three days. In general, it is not a good idea to lift weights every day unless you vary the muscle groups you are working with each day. In one study on weight-lifting and depression, the women lifted weights that were 45–87 per cent as heavy as the maximum they could lift at one time. The women who lifted weights closer to the top end of this range saw the greatest benefits. These women lifted weights three days a week for 10 weeks, gradually increasing the amount of weight they lifted at each session.

Weight-lifting requires training in order to do it safely and properly, so you will need to take a few classes at a local gym, sports club or recreation centre. When aerobics and weight-lifting are alternated, you will have a really comprehensive training regime designed to benefit the cardiovascular system, muscles, tendons, ligaments and bones. Regular weight-bearing exercise is also helpful in preventing osteoporosis.

Too much exercise

Whilst the vast majority of people with depression will benefit from doing more exercise, there are a few for whom it could be harmful. According to Chinese medical theory, all activity entails a consumption of yin by yang. If someone is constitutionally deficient in yin, or if circumstances such as ageing, persistent illness, extreme blood loss, excessive births or lactation have depleted their yin, too much exercise or physical activity can worsen the situation. This condition is can be seen in women with thin bodily constitutions who overexercise, such as professional athletes, or in women who suffer from anorexia and bulimia.

Body fat in Chinese medicine is considered to be yin. So someone who is very thinly built tends to have less yin to start off with. If the body fat is further reduced through exercise, it may become so insufficient that yin can no longer control yang. In women, such a deficiency of yin blood due to too much exercise usually manifests first as cessation of menstruation, or amenorrhoea. It is also possible for the use of drugs, especially amphetamines or 'speed', and eating disorders such as anorexia and bulimia, to result in an overconsumption of yin. This can lead to amenorrhoea, increased mental agitation and insomnia. In the case of bulimia, although they are eating the person is not getting sufficient yin nourishment as they are bingeing and purging.

You will know that the amount of exercise you do is correct if you feel refreshed and invigorated a couple of hours after the exercise is over. If you notice that you feel even more fatigued or nervous and jittery or if exercise during the day leads to night sweats and insomnia at night, then you need to reduce your level of exercise.

DEEP RELAXATION

As we have seen, depression is very often associated with liver depression qi stagnation. This condition arises because of emotional upset, frustration and stress. When we have liver depression qi stagnation that persists for a long time it creates heat, which in turn consumes the yin of the body (heat and fire are considered to be yang). This heat or fire rises in the body and disturbs the heart spirit, causing anxiety and agitation. We will feel irritable, easily angered and tense. According to Chinese medicine, every emotion or thought effects the flow of qi. Anger in particular makes the qi flow upwards. We can therefore influence the flow of qi by changing our thoughts and emotions. That is why deep relaxation is so important in helping to control depression. Deep relaxation needs to involve the body as well as the mind.

Guided deep relaxation tapes

An effective way to practise such mental and physical deep relaxation is to listen to a daily, guided, progressive, deep relaxation audiotape. It is guided in the sense that a narrator on the tape leads you through the process of deep relaxation. These tapes normally lead you to relax the body in a progressive manner, first relaxing one part and then moving on to another.

There are many such tapes available, usually sold in health food shops or good bookshops. Choose several tapes so that you won't get too bored, listening to the same one. When looking for a good relaxation tape, firstly ensure that the tape is a guided tape and not a subliminal relaxation tape. Subliminal tapes usually have music, and any instructions to relax are given so quietly that they are not consciously heard. Although such tapes can help you feel relaxed when you use them, ultimately they do not teach you how to relax as a skill that you can then consciously practise. Secondly, make sure the tape starts from the top of the body and works downwards. This is because anger makes the qi go upwards in the body; frustration and anger due to liver depression qi stagnation means there is already too much qi rising upwards in the body. This depressed qi needs not only to be moved but to be moved downwards. Thirdly, make sure the tape instructs you to relax your physical body. If you do not relax all your muscles or sinews, the qi cannot flow freely and the liver cannot be coursed. The tape will not be as beneficial if you don't relax your muscles. Finally, try to make sure the tape instructs you to let your breath go with each exhalation. One of the symptoms of liver depression is a stuffy feeling in the chest, which we then unconsciously try to relieve by sighing. Letting each exhalation go completely helps the lungs push the qi downwards.

The importance of daily practice

One of the authors was once taken on a field trip to a hospital clinic where they were using deep relaxation as a therapy with patients with high blood pressure, heart disease, stroke, migraines and insomnia. The doctors at this clinic produced various graphs plotting their research data on how such daily, progressive, deep relaxation can regulate the blood pressure and body temperature and improve the appetite, digestion, elimination, sleep, energy and mood. One of the things they said has stuck with him for 15 years: 'Small results in 100 days, big results in 1,000.' This means that if one does such daily, progressive, deep relaxation every single day for 100 days, one will definitely experience certain results. What are these 'small' results? They are improvements in all the parameters listed above, i.e. blood pressure, body temperature, appetite, digestion, elimination, sleep, energy and mood. The 'big' results experienced in 1,000 days of practice are more fundamental. They really are about a change in how one reacts to stress and are much more permanent.

What these doctors in Shanghai stressed, which the author has also experienced both personally and with patients, is that the effects of this relaxation are cumulative, meaning that the longer one can practise this routine on a consistent daily basis, the greater and more lasting the effects will be.

It is vitally important to do such dguided, progressive, deep relaxation on a daily basis for at the very least three months and ideally for three years. If you achieved this goal then you would see every parameter of health and well-being improve. If you do this kind of deep relaxation sporadically, missing a day here and there, it will have some benefit, but it will not have the marked, cumulative therapeutic effects which are possible.

The real test

Doing a daily, deep relaxation regime is only practice, however. It's like hitting tennis balls against a wall or hitting a bucket of balls at a driving range: it's not the real thing. The real purpose of a daily deep relaxation regime is not just to relieve the immediate stress and strain but to learn a new skill, a new way to react to stress. The ultimate goal is to recondition how you react in stressful situations, learning how to breathe out and relax your muscles rather than holding your breath and tensing your muscles. This is the real test, the game of life. Remember: 'Small results in 100 days, big results in 1,000.'

SIMPLE HOME REMEDIES FOR DEPRESSION

By changing your diet, getting adequate exercise and altering how you deal with stress in a fundamental way you will significantly improve your depression. These lifestyle changes are probably the most important things that you could do for yourself. In this chapter we will look at some simple home remedies based on Chinese medicine, which you may find useful to help relieve some of the symptoms of depression.

CHINESE AROMATHERAPY

Although aromatherapy has been a major part of professionally practised Chinese medicine for almost 1,000 years, there is a simple aromatherapy treatment that one can do at home which can help alleviate irritability, depression, nervousness, anxiety and insomnia.

An ingredient often used in Asian incense is Lignum Aquilariae Agallochae (eaglewood). The Chinese name for it is *Chen Xiang,* which means 'sinking fragrance'. In Chinese medicine, Aquilaria is classified as a qi-rectifying medicinal. When used as a boiled decoction or 'tea', Aquilaria stops pain and promotes the movement of the qi in a downward direction in the body. The reason it is called sinking fragrance probably has to do with this ability to move the qi downwards. When it is burnt as a medicinal incense it is very calming and soothing.

You should be able to buy this herb from specialist Chinese herbal suppliers or shops. The powdered variety is best but if this is not available then you can powder your own in a coffee grinder or just use the herb in small pieces. You will also need to buy some incense charcoal. To carry out the treatment, light an incense charcoal in an inflammable dish and put a few small pinches of the Aquilaria on it. As the smoke rises inhale deeply. This treatment can be done on an as needed basis or, if suffering from depression, repeat it at least three times a week. It will help with restlessness, nervousness, anxiety and irritability.

CHINESE SELF-MASSAGE

The self-massage regime below is specifically designed as a home remedy for depression. For further Chinese self-massage regimes, we recommend Fan Ya-li's *Chinese Self-massage Therapy: The Easy Way to Health* (see page 170).

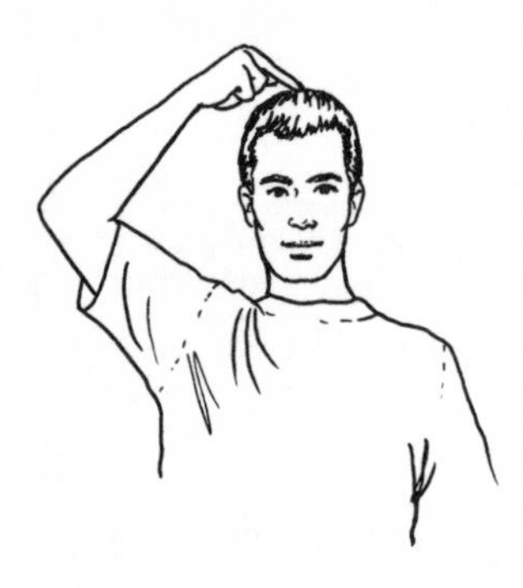

1. Begin by pressing and kneading the very centre and top of the skull. This is acupoint *Bai Hui* (Governing vessel 20). It is the most yang point in the body and is the meeting place of all the yang channels and vessels. It is especially useful for calming the spirit, soothing the liver and subduing hyperactive yang. Do this approximately 100 times.

2. With the fingertips of both hands, knead the acupoint located at the inner ends of the eyebrows. This area corresponds to the point *Zhan Zhu* (Bladder 2). It is the place where the yang qi travelling up a channel known as the *yang qiao mai* connects with the yin *qiao mai* which leads downwards. Knead this area approximately 30 times.

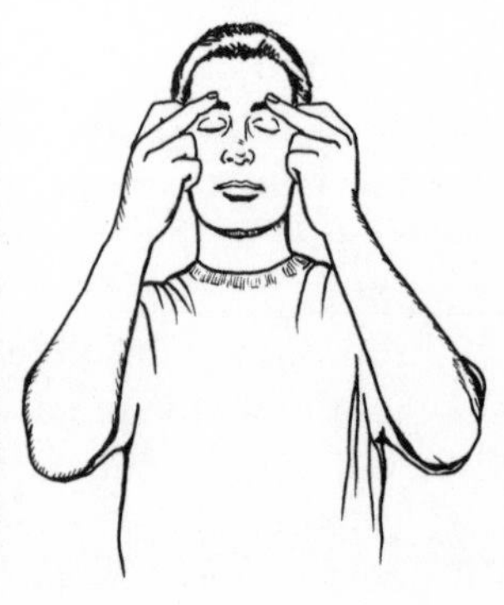

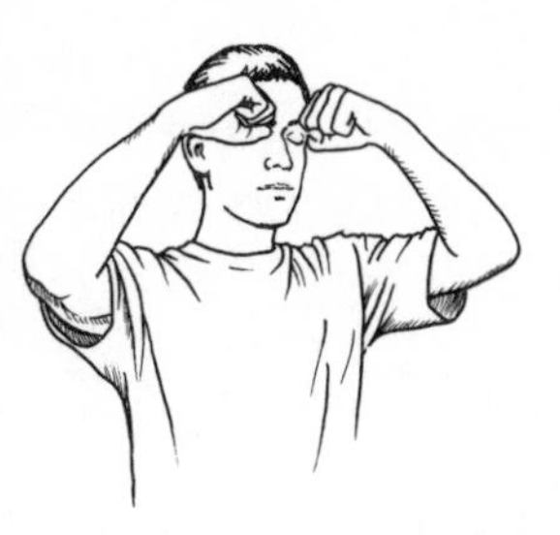

3. With the index fingers and thumbs, wipe the upper edge of the eye bone and then the lower edge. Work from the inner corners of the eyes to the outer corners. This helps move the yang qi in the eyes downwards and keeps it from becoming congested. Repeat this 20–30 times.

4. Rub the palms of the hands vigorously together until they feel warm. Then place these warm palms over both eyes. Cover the eyes thus for 30–60 seconds and then lightly rub the closed eyes approximately 10 times.

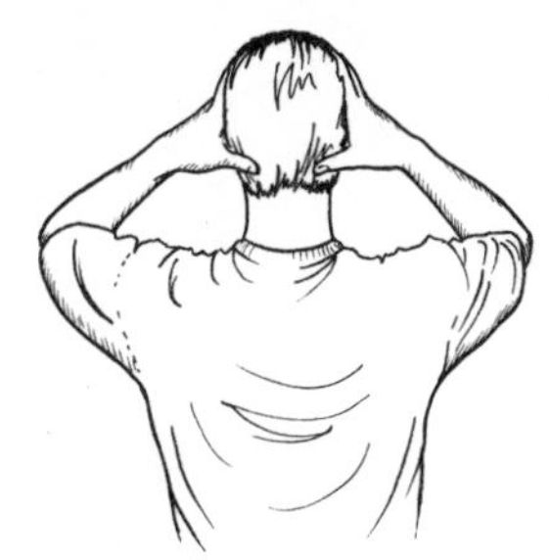

5. Press and knead the acupoint *Feng Chi* (Governing vessel 20) with the thumbs. This point is located in the depression between the mastoid process, the bone behind the ear and the strap muscles that connect at the base of the skull. The point is located approximately 2.5 cm/1 in within the hairline on most people. It is a point which people often find themselves instinctively massaging when they have a tension head or stiff neck. Repeat 30–50 times, massaging both points with both hands at the same time.

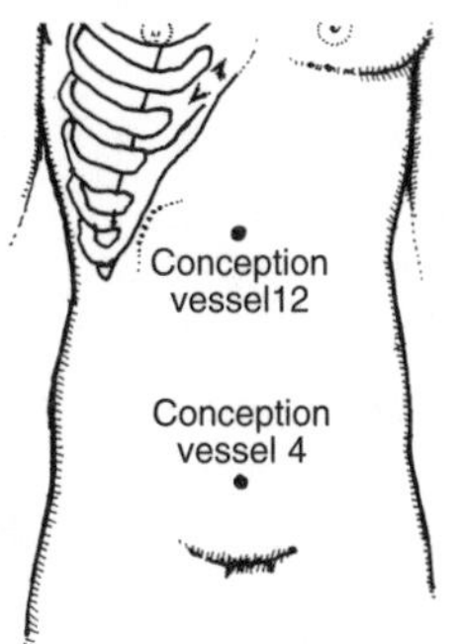

6. Rub circles around the centre of the upper and the lower abdomen. The point in the middle of the upper abdomen is called *Zhong Wan* (Conception vessel 12). The point in the centre of the lower abdomen is called *Guan Yuan* (Conception vessel 4). Rub these first clockwise and then anticlockwise approximately 100 times each point in each direction.

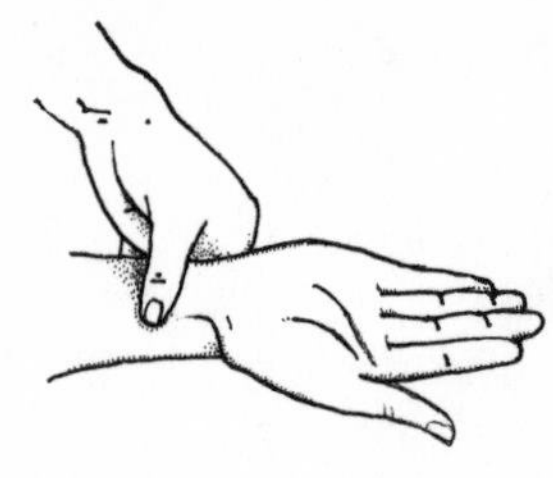

7. Press and knead the acupoint *Nei Guan* (Pericardium 6). This point is located on the inner side of the forearm in between the two tendons. It is located approximately 4 cm/1½ in upwards from the wrist. First press and knead one thumb and then press and knead with the other. Repeat approximately 30–50 times on each side. This point helps soothe the liver, regulate the qi and quiet the spirit.

8. Press and knead the point *Shen Men* (Heart 7). This is located on the inner side of the forearm at the crease of the wrist right below the base of the little finger. Massage the points on both wrists 30–50 times each. This point clears heat from the heart and quiets the spirit.

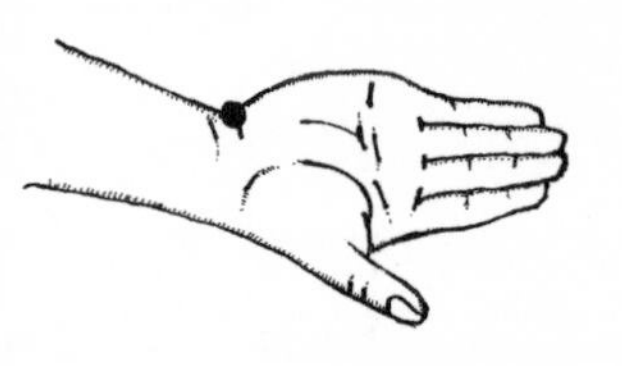

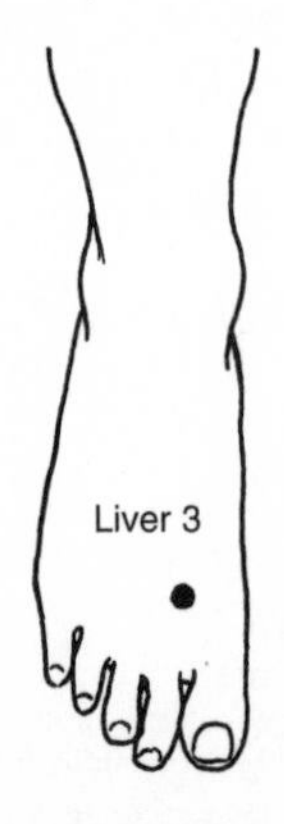

9. Press and knead the point *He Gu* (Large intestine 4). This point is located on the top of the hand, between the thumb and the index finger; at the highest spot of the muscle when the thumb and index finger are brought close together. Choose the hand on one side and then move contralaterally to the opposite foot. Here on the foot press and knead *Tai Chong* (Liver 3) located on the top of the foot between the first and second toes, about 5 cm/2 in away from the margin of the web towards the body. Do *Tai Chong* on the other foot and then move to do *He Gu* on the other hand. This will help open the Four Gates.

10. Knead and press *Zu San Li* (Stomach 36). This point is located 8 cm/3 in below the lower, outside edge of the kneecap when the leg is bent. It is located in a depression between the muscles of the lower leg. Massage this point 30–50 times on each side. This point regulates the qi and leads counterflowing yang qi downwards.

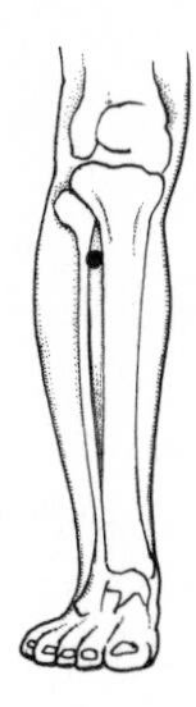

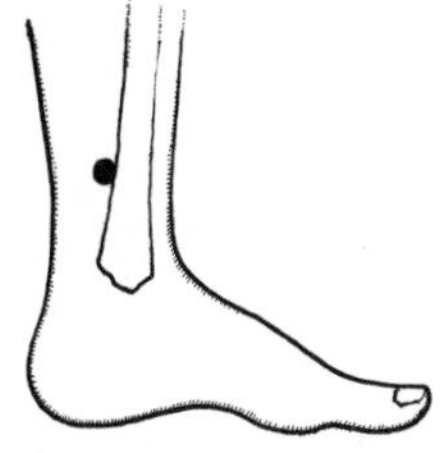

11. Follow this by pressing and kneading *San Yin Jiao* (Spleen 6). This point is located 7.5 cm/3 in above the tip of the inner ankle bone on the back side of the lower leg bone. It is the meeting place of the liver, spleen and kidney channels. It is very effective for stimulating the production of yin blood in the body, which can then control the yang qi.

12. Finally, rub the depression just behind and to the side of the ball of the foot. This point is called *Yong Quan* (Kidney 1). This is considered to be the most yin point of the body in relation to *Bai Hui* (Governing vessel 20), which is the most yang. Stimulating this point helps to lead counterflowing yang qi back down to its lower source. Rub this point with the palm of the opposite hand until it feels hot. Repeat this on the other foot.

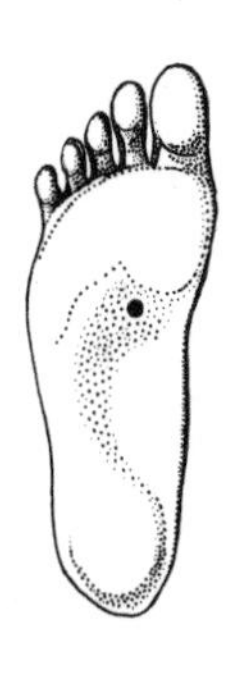

This self-massage regime should take between 20–30 minutes. It should ideally be done every evening just before bed. When doing each massage manipulation it is helpful to try to focus calmly on the physical sensations under your hands and not let your mind wander to your day's worries and stresses.

SEVEN STAR HAMMERING

A seven star hammer is a small hammer or mallet with seven small needles embedded in its head. This is one way to stimulate acupuncture points without inserting a needle into the body, and is also an excellent method for moving congested qi. Seven star hammers can be useful for those who are frightened of needles and for children, as well as for home therapy treatment. When the points to be stimulated are located on the front of the body you may do the treatment yourself. You will, however, need to get someone to assist if the points are located on the back of the body.

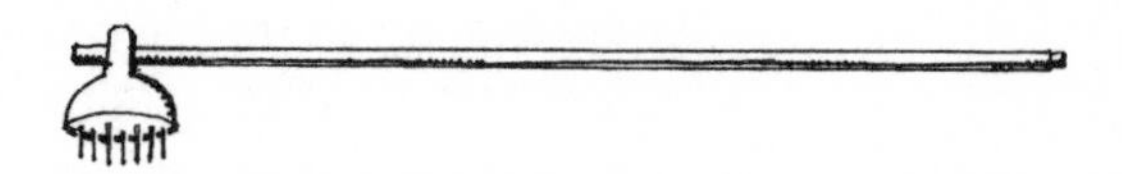

At least part of this seven star treatment for depression will require an assistant or helper. Firstly, disinfect all the areas of the skin that are going to be tapped. Begin by lightly tapping on the back of the neck. Lightly tap all along the centre of the spine on the neck, as well as up and down the strap muscles to either side of the spinal column. Then lightly tap acupoints *Feng Chi* (Gall bladder 20). The location of these points behind the mastoid processes behind the ears has been described in the section on Chinese self-massage (see page 115) If you suffer from depressive heat with red eyes, red face, headache and/or dizziness, you can tap until the points bleed a very small amount. This helps drain heat or fire from the upper body. Otherwise tap until the skin is simply flushed red.

Next, tap all over the sacrum lightly until it turns a light red colour.

Then tap the centre of the sternum lightly; there is a point in the midline of the sternum, midway between the two nipples. This point, *Shan Zhong* (Conception vessel 17), opens up the chest, relieves anxiety and irritability and has a calming but invigorating effect. At the sides of the body, tap on the line that extends from under the armpit to the space between the fifth and sixth ribs (count the intercostal spaces between the ribs next to the sternum and then follow it around). The point is about 12 cm/5 in below the armpit and corresponds to the point *Da Bao* (Spleen 21), which opens up the chest, relaxes the diaphragm and helps circulate stagnant qi in the whole thoracic region.

Follow this by tapping *Nei Guan* (Pericardium 6), *Shen Men* (Heart 7) and *San Yin Jiao* (Spleen 6), in that order. Then tap *He Gu* (Large intestine 4) and *Tai Chong* (Liver 3) on opposite sides. The locations of these five points have also been given under the section on Chinese self-massage (see pages 114–17).

If you have a headache (particularly one that is due to ascendant hyperactivity of liver yang), tap gently over both temples. If the headache is severe, tap till there is a very small amount of bleeding.

If there is any bleeding when you use the seven star hammer, wipe the area with a cotton swab moistened in alcohol or hydrogen peroxide. Then take a dry cotton wool ball and press the area. Between treatments, soak the seven star hammer in alcohol or hydrogen peroxide. In order to prevent infection always use your own personal hammer – do not share with anyone else.

THREAD MOXIBUSTION

Thread moxibustion involves burning extremely tiny cones or 'threads' of a dried herb, Folium Artemisae Argyii *(Aiye)*, also known as Oriental mugwort, directly on top of certain chosen points. When done correctly, this is a very simple and effective way of adding yang qi to the body without causing a burn or scar. Since most people with depression have at least some element of spleen qi and possible kidney yang vacuity, so adding yang qi to the body may be very beneficial. If you suffer from depressive heat or yin vacuity, you will need to seek professional advice before trying this self-treatment as the heat from the moxa may aggravate your condition.

To do thread moxibustion, you will require the finest quality or grade of Japanese moxa. Pinch off a very small amount of this loose moxa and roll it lightly between the thumb and forefinger. You are aiming to make a loose, very thin thread of moxa, smaller than a grain of rice. It is important that this thread is not too large or too tightly wrapped.

Next, rub a very thin film of Tiger Balm or Temple of Heaven Balm on the point to be treated. These are camphorated Chinese medical salves, which are widely available. Ensure that the salve is very thinly or sparingly applied. If these Chinese medicated salves are not available, then wipe the point with a tiny amount of vegetable oil or even just wet the point with water. Stand the thread of moxa up perpendicularly directly on the point. The oil, balm or water should provide enough stickiness to make the thread stand on end. Light the thread with a thin, burning incense stick, sometimes called an akabane stick. As the thread burns down towards the skin, you will feel it get warm and then hot. Immediately remove the burning thread as soon as you feel some heat. Do not burn yourself. It is better to pull the thread off too soon than too late. If you do burn yourself, apply some lavender aromatherapy oil directly on the burn.

Having removed the burning thread and extinguished it between your two fingers, repeat this process again. To speed up the process you can roll a number of threads before starting the treatment. Each time the thread burns down close to the skin, pinch it off the skin and extinguish it before it starts to burn you. If you do this correctly, your skin will get red and hot to the touch but you will not raise a blister. As the skin texture may vary from person to person it is best to start out with three or four threads to see how you react. Increase the number of threads to nine to 12 threads per treatment.

This treatment is especially effective for women in their late 30s and throughout their 40s, whose spleen and kidney yang qi has already weakened, or in older people of both sexes. This treatment adds yang qi to the body, it fortifies the spleen and invigorates the kidneys, warming yang and boosting the qi. It is best to do this treatment daily for a number of days. This can be a very beneficial home therapy for women who suffer from PMS where there are other symptoms involved like premenstrual fatigue, loose stools, cold hands and feet, low or no libido and lower back or knee pain accompanied by frequent night-time urination (which is generally copious and clear). We recommend beginning this moxibustion just before ovulation, around day 10 in the cycle. It should then be repeated every day up to the first day of the period and then suspended. It can be done for several months in a row, but shouldn't be done on a continual daily basis throughout the year.

There are three points that should be treated with this supplementing technique. These are:

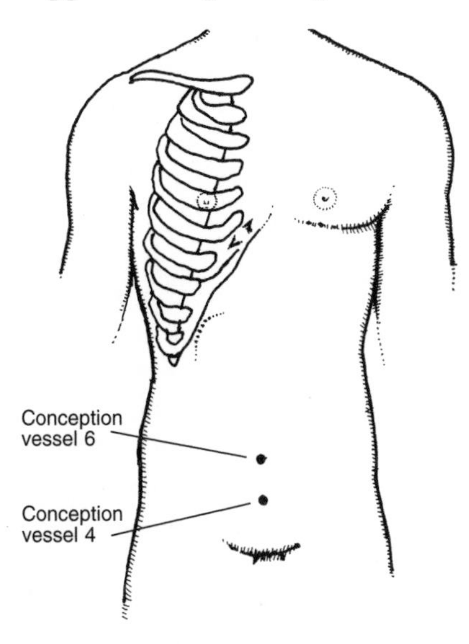

Qi Hai
(Conception vessel 6)
Guan Yuan
(Conception vessel 4)
Zu San Li
(Stomach 36)

Qi Hai is located on the midline of the body, two finger-widths below the navel. *Guan Yuan* is also located on the midline of the lower abdomen, four finger-widths below the navel.

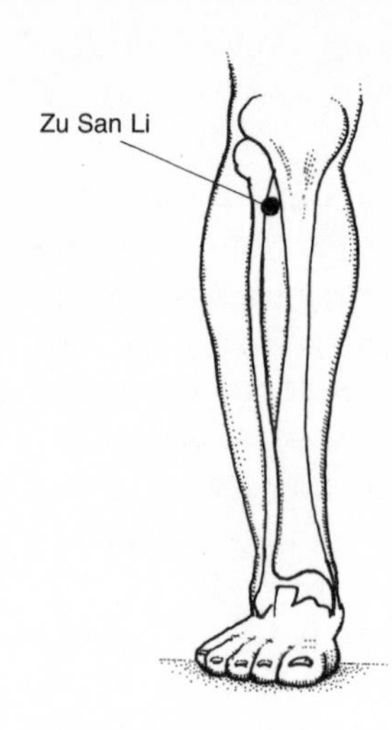

Zu San Li is located four finger-widths below the lower edge of the kneecap between the tibia and fibula on the outside edge of the lower leg. However, we highly recommend visiting a professional acupuncturist so that they can teach you how to do this technique safely and effectively, and show you how to locate these three points accurately.

In Chinese medicine, this technique is considered to promote longevity and health preservation. It is excellent for those people whose yang qi has already begun to decline due to the inevitable ageing process. It may not be beneficial for someone with ascension of hyperactive liver yang, liver fire or depressive liver heat, as more heat might aggravate the situation. It is best done starting from the topmost point and moving down the body.

There is another method of stimulating the acupuncture points with warmth, which is very simple and easily done. Take a card and poke a small hole in it. Place the card over the point to be stimulated and use a hairdryer to blow warm air on the point. This should feel pleasantly warm, not uncomfortably hot.

If there is any doubt about whether these techniques are appropriate for you, please seek professional advice from a practitioner of Chinese medicine.

FLOWER THERAPY

The beauty of flowers is a wonderful way to bring joy into your life. Joy is so important because it is such a healing emotion – remember how we said earlier that every emotion or thought effects the flow of qi in the body. This is particularly beneficial in the case of depression. Buying yourself a bunch of flowers can simply make you feel better about yourself.

Another important aspect of flowers is their fragrance. Chrysanthemums, for example, have a relaxing and calming fragrance. Roses have a smell that is said to 'quicken the blood'. According to Chinese herbal medicine, flowers that are used to calm the spirit are: lily, narcissus, lotus, orchid and jasmine. Taking a sniff of a bouquet of flowers is a great way of releasing pent-up tensions in the chest.

LIGHT THERAPY

Light therapy, heliotherapy or sunbathing is a health preservation and longevity practice according to Chinese medicine. Sunlight is considered to be the most essential yang qi in nature. Li Shi-zhen, one of the most famous Chinese doctors of the late Ming dynasty (1368–1644 AD), wrote, '*Tai yang* (a name for the sun) is true fire.' He pointed out, 'Without fire, heaven is not able to engender things and without fire, people are not able to live.' Since the back of the body is relatively yang (as compared to the front which is more yin), exposing the back to sunlight is a good way of increasing our yang qi.

As we have seen above, the yang qi begins to decline in most women by around 35 years of age. After a woman has reached the age of 35 symptoms such as premenstrual fatigue, loose stools, lack of strength, poor memory, lack of concentration, poor co-ordination, decline in or lack of libido, lower back and knee pain and weakness, increased night-time urination and cold hands and feet are due to this decline, firstly in the yang qi of the spleen and later in the yang qi of both the spleen and kidneys. The spleen qi and kidney yang decline in both sexes as part of the ageing process. This decline in yang qi may play a role in depression in older people. This means that sunbathing can help supplement the yang qi of the body, strengthening the spleen and/or kidneys.

Yang qi is considered to be the motivating force that pushes the qi. Increasing the yang qi can move stagnation and help resolve depression. Cao Ting-dong, a famous doctor of the Ch'ing dynasty (1644–1911 AD), wrote 'Sitting with the back exposed directly to the sun, the back may get warmed. This is able to make the entire body harmonious and smoothly flowing. The sun is the essence of *tai yang* and its light strengthens the yang qi of the human body.'

In Chinese medicine, whenever the words 'harmonious' and 'smoothly flowing' are used together, they refer to the flow of qi and blood. So sunbathing can help course the liver and rectify the qi as well as fortify the spleen and invigorate the kidneys.

We now know that overexposure to the sun can cause skin cancer, so it is important to take care with sunbathing and not to burn. According to Chinese medicine, sunbathing should be done between the hours of 8 and10 a.m. You should only sunbathe between 11 a.m. and 1 p.m. in winter in temperate, not tropical, latitudes. Wearing a sunscreen of SPF 15 or higher will not effect the therapeutic warming effects of sunbathing from a Chinese medical point of view.

It is interesting to note that some Western researchers are coming to understand that exposure to light does play a role in premenstrual syndrome (PMS) and seasonal affective disorder (SAD). Both these conditions may affect depression.

CHINESE HERBAL REMEDIES

In this next section we will give you some recipes that you can make at home in the form of wines, teas and porridges. As with all Chinese herbs we strongly recommend that you seek professional guidance with regard to their usage. Should you choose to try one of these recipes and notice any unwanted side-effects, stop taking it immediately and seek professional advice.

Chinese medicinal wines

Chinese medicinal wines are part of Chinese dietary therapy. They make use of the special characteristics of alcohol as well as a few Chinese herbs or medicinals. Although alcohol is hot and can inflame yang heat, especially liver heat, it has the ability to move depressed qi and static blood. It can also speed up and increase the medicinal effects of herbs in the body. We recommend that you use caution should you try these recipes to improve symptoms of depression.

For liver depression with chest oppression, irritability and insomnia:

50 g/2 oz Flos Albizziae Julibrissinis *(He Huan Pi)*
50 g/2 oz Flos Rosae Rugosae *(Mei Gui Hua)*
50 g/2 oz Caulis Polygoni Multiflori *(Ye Jiao Teng)*

Soak in 1.2 litres/2 pts of either brandy or vodka for one month. Strain off the dregs and drink 25–50 ml/1½–3 tbsp of the liquid before or after dinner.

For liver depression with chest oppression, distension and pain in the sides of the ribs, epigastric aching and pain or breast distension and pain, soak 120 g/4½ oz Rhizoma Cyperi Rotundi *(Xiang Fu)* in 1.2 litres/2 pts of vodka or brandy for one month, strain off the dregs and take 15 ml of the liquid. Repeat throughout the day. Do not use this formula if there are signs of heat such as red eyes, red face, actual anger or a red tongue with yellow fur.

For liver depression causing dizziness, headache or one-sided headache, soak 200 g/7 oz Fructus Viticis *(Man Jing Zi)* in 1.2 litres/2 pts of brandy or vodka for one month. Strain off the dregs and drink 25 ml/1½ tbsp or so of the remaining liquid at the time of the dizziness or headache.

A slightly more elaborate formula for the same condition consists of:

60 g/2 oz Fructus Viticis *(Man Jing Zi)*
30 g/1 oz Flos Chrysanthemi Morifolii *(Ju Hua)*

30 g/1 oz Radix Ligustici Wallichii *(Chuan Xiong)*
30 g/1 oz Radix Ledebouriellae Divaricatae *(Fang Feng)*
30 g/1 oz Herba Menthae Haplocalycis *(Bo He)*

Make and take the same way as the preceding 'wine'. This second formula can be cautiously tried even if there are signs and symptoms of depressive heat.

For depressive liver heat with red eyes, headache and dizziness, soak 125 g/4¾ oz Flos Chrysanthemi Morifolii *(Ju Hua)* in 1.2 litres/2 pts of brandy or vodka for one month. Strain off the dregs and drink 25 ml/1½ tbsp of the remaining liquid before or after dinner.

For heart blood-spleen qi vacuity depression, try either of two home-made Chinese medicinal wines. The first is made by placing 150 g/5 oz white ginseng (Radix Panacis Ginseng, *Ren Shen*) in 1.2 litres/2 pts of brandy for one to two months. Then strain off the dregs and take 25–50 ml/1½–3 tbsp of the remaining liquid before or after dinner. Do not use this wine if you display the signs and symptoms of depressive liver heat affecting the head and face. Alternatively, use 150 g/5 oz Arillus Euphoriae Longanae *(Long Yan Rou)* steeped in 1.2 litres/2 pts sake. Drink 25–50 ml/1½–3 tbsp before or after dinner each evening. Do not take this latter wine if you suffer from constipation.

For depression due to phlegm blocking or confounding the portals of the heart, soak 120 g/4½ oz Rhizoma Acori Graminei *(Shi Chang Pu)* in 1.2 litres/2 pts of vodka for three to five days. Then take 10–20 ml/2–4 tsp of the resulting medicinal wine three times a day on an empty stomach.

These are only a few of the Chinese medicinal wines and elixirs that can be made and used at home for the treatment of depression. More information on Chinese medicinal wines may be found in *Chinese Medical Wines and Elixirs* (see page 156).

Chinese medicinal porridges

Like the Chinese medicinal wines discussed above, Chinese medicinal porridges are a specialised part of Chinese dietary therapy. Porridges are very easily digestible since they they are eaten when already cooked and warm, they are a particularly good way of eating nutritious but possibly indigestible grains. When Chinese medicinals are cooked together with grains in the form of a porridge, you have a high-powered and easily assimilated nutritious 'health food' of the first order.

For liver depression qi stagnation pattern of depression, cook 50 g/2 oz white rice with 10 g/¼ oz Pericarpium Citri Reticulatae Viride *(Qing Pi)*. Eat this once a day. Another possibility is to cook 5 g Flos Pruni (i.e. plum flowers) with 100 g/4 oz white rice in enough water to make a thin porridge or gruel.

For spleen qi vacuity with pronounced fatigue, cook 30 g/1 oz Radix Astragali Membranacei *(Huang Qi)* with 6 g Pericarpium Citri Reticulatae *(Chen Pi)* in 600 ml/1 pt water for 20 minutes. Strain off the dregs and then use the resulting medicinal 'tea' to cook 50 g/2 oz white rice. Another possibility for treating spleen qi vacuity fatigue and lack of strength is to take 3g powdered Radix Panacis Ginseng *(Ren Shen)* and cook this with 100 g/4 oz white rice in water. A third option is to take 5 g ginseng and 20 g/¾ oz powdered Sclerotium Poriae Cocos *(Fu Ling)* and cook this with 60 g/ 4¼ oz white rice in water. During the last 5–7 minutes of cooking, add a couple of slices of fresh ginger. If you cannot find ginseng, you can use 30 g/1 oz Radix Codonopsitis Pilosulae *(Dang Shen)* cooked with 50 g/2 oz white rice in water. Remove the codonopsis and eat the resulting porridge.

For heart blood–spleen qi vacuity depression, cook 100 g/ 4 oz white rice with 50 g/2 oz Semen Coicis Lachrymajobi *(Yi Yi Ren)* and 10 red dates (Fructus Zizyphi Jujubae, *Da Zao)*. Another alternative is to cook 100 g/4 oz white rice in chicken broth with 10 red dates and eat this for dinner every evening for a few days.

For depression accompanied by insomnia and anxiety due to blood and yin vacuity, use 15 g/½ oz Semen Biota Orientalis *(Bai Zi Ren)* or Semen Zizyphi Spinosae *(Suan Zao Ren)* with 100 g/4 oz white rice and again cook with enough water to make a thin porridge or gruel. Alternatively, simply eat cream of wheat every evening before bed instead of dessert.

For depression accompanied by phlegm confounding or blocking the portals of the heart, try cooking 5 g powdered Rhizoma Acori Graminei *(Shi Chang Pu)* with 50 g/2 oz white rice in water.

For numerous other Chinese medicinal porridge formulae for depression, see *The Book of Jook: Chinese Medicinal Porridges: A Healthy Alternative to the Typical Western Breakfast* (see page 156).

Chinese medicinal teas

Chinese herbal teas generally consist of one or two Chinese herbal medicinals, which are made into a tea and consumed throughout the day. Chinese medicinal teas are usually simpler to prepare and taste better than multi-ingredient, professionally prescribed decoctions. They can be used in addition to professionally prescribed Chinese herbs or as an adjunct to acupuncture or other Chinese therapies for depression.

For liver depression qi stagnation, take 100–150 g/4–6 oz fresh plums and add to 320 ml/11 fl oz water in a pot and boil for three minutes. Then add 2 g green tea and 25 g/1 oz honey and steep for 10 minutes. Take one dose in the morning and another dose in the evening. This formula is especially effective for abdominal distension and epigastric oppression associated with liver depression. Another simple tea for liver depression qi stagnation can be made by boiling 25 g/1 oz each Fructus Immaturus Citri Aurantii *(Zhi Shi)* and Pericarpium Citri Reticulatae *(Chen Pi)* in water for several minutes. Then add 2 g green tea and steep for 10 minutes. Drink the resulting tea any time during the day. Another tea which may be useful for this condition of liver depression qi stagnation may be made by taking 10 g Tuber Curcumae *(Yu Jin)*, i.e. turmeric, and boiling it in 1 litre/1¾ pts water with 5 g Radix Glycyrrhizae *(Gan Cao)*, i.e. liquorice. Then add 2 g green tea and a little honey to taste. Drink this throughout the day.

For liver depression/depressive heat, boil 30 g/1 oz each green tea and Fructus Gardeniae Jasminoidis *(Shan Zhi Zi)* in 1.2 litres/2 pts water and boil until the liquid is reduced by half. Strain off the dregs and drink one cup of this liquid in the morning and another in the evening. Or take 15 g/½ oz Flos Chrysanthemi Morifolii *(Ju Hua)* and steep this with 2 g green tea in boiling water for 10 minutes. Drink the tea throughout the day. In addition, jasmine tea purchased at Asian speciality food shops, is a good background beverage for those with liver depression with or without heat.

For spleen vacuity fatigue and lack of strength, boil 8 g Radix Panacis Ginseng *(Ren Shen)* for an hour or more in 250 ml/8 fl oz water. Drink this as a tea throughout the day. Asian speciality food stores often sell small porcelain ginseng cookers. These are lidded cups meant to be placed in a pan of water to create a small double-cooker. Basically, the longer you cook ginseng, the more you get out of it. As a substitute for ginseng, you can use double the amount of Radix Codonopsitis Pilosulae *(Dang Shen)*. Do not use ginseng if you suffer from hypertension or high blood pressure. In our clinical experience, it is much more common to find depression and chronic fatigue occurring in those with hypotension or low blood pressure.

If you suffer from spleen qi and heart blood vacuity, you can try making a tea from 9 g Radix Pseudostellariae *(Tai Zi Shen)* and 15 g/½ oz Semen Levis Tritici Aestivi *(Fu Xiao Mai)*. Place both of these ingredients in a vacuum flask and steep in boiling water for 20 minutes. Then drink as a tea throughout the day. Alternatively, you can use 5–10 pieces of Arillus Euphoriae Longanae *(Long Yan Rou)*. Place these dried fruits in a double boiler or pressure cooker and steam thoroughly. Then put them in a teacup and steep in boiling water for 10 minutes. Drink the resulting liquid as a tea. Another possibility is to boil 10 pieces of Fructus Zizyphi Jujubae *(Da Zao)* in water until the fruit is thoroughly cooked and completely soft. Then use the resulting liquid to steep 5 g green tea. Drink this as a tea any time throughout the day.

For depression due to heart yin and blood vacuity, grind 15 g/½ oz Semen Biotae Orientalis *(Bai Zi Ren)* into pieces. Boil with water for 10 minutes and add honey to taste. Drink either before or after dinner. Or boil 15 g/½ oz Fructus Mori Albi *(Sang Zhen)* in water. Strain off the dregs and drink the resulting liquid throughout the day. This dose is for a one-day supply. Another option is to grind into powder equal amounts of Fructus Schisandrae Chinensis *(Wu Wei Zi)* and Fructus Lycii Chinensis *(Gou Qi Zi)*. Then use 5 g of this powder steeped in boiling water for 10 minutes as a tea throughout the day. Or you may use 9 g Semen Zizyphi Spinosae *(Suan Zao Ren)*. Pound these into pieces, steep in boiling water for 10 minutes and drink throughout the day.

For phlegm obstruction with liver depression/depressive heat, grind 6 g Rhizoma Acori Graminei *(Shi Chang Pu)*, 6 g Flos Jasmini *(Mo Li Hua)*, and 10 g green tea into coarse powder. Soak some of this powder in boiling water and drink as a tea any time of the day. (You can also use jasmine tea bought at an Asian speciality food shop.) For another formula for phlegm obstruction disturbing the heart spirit but without the heat, boil 10 g Dens Draconis *(Long Chi)* in water for 10 minutes. Then add 3 g Rhizoma Acori Graminei *(Shi Chang Pu)* and continue boiling for another 10–15 minutes. Strain off the dregs and drink the liquid any time of the day. The doses given are for one day's supply.

For fire disturbing the heart spirit characterised by restlessness and insomnia, vexation and agitation, a red tongue tip, sores on the tip of the tongue and heart palpitations, boil 60 g/2½ oz each Medulla Junci Effusi *(Deng*

Xin Cao) and Folium Lophatheri Gracilis *(Dan Zhu Ye)*. Strain off the dregs and drink the resulting tea warm at any time of the day. This dose is a one-day supply.

For more information on books about Chinese medicinal teas, see page 156.

CREATING A PERSONAL REGIME

It is not necessary to do all these home treatments if you are suffering from depression. Choose several of them that appeal to you and are manageable. The more severe your depression, the more support you are likely to need. It is best to make sure you are using the three 'free' therapies and then add these home remedies depending on what you can best manage.

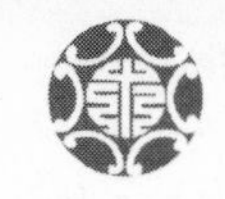

ADDITIONAL SUGGESTIONS FROM CLINICAL EXPERIENCE

LETTING NEGATIVE THOUGHTS AND FEELINGS BE

Some people who are experiencing a depressive episode are not totally clear about the issues that precipitated the depression in the first place. Others may understand the causes and triggering factors but are still unable to cut through the experience of being depressed.

We may use up a great deal of energy to fight the anger, frustration, disappointment and exhaustion that frequently underlie depression. We react to uncomfortable feelings in much the same way as we react to pain. We constrict, close down and squeeze in, trying to protect ourselves from the hurt. This is why we recommended deep relaxation therapy earlier in the book and why this deep relaxation needs to be somatic (bodily) relaxation and not just mental relaxation. Our mental attitude can however be very important. We may need to develop an ability simply to let things be as they are. Fighting with our thoughts and emotions does not ultimately help the situation and may even exacerbate it. If we allow our emotions and thoughts the space to be as they are, they will eventually transform into something else.

According to Asian philosophy, whether it is Buddhism, Confucianism or Taoism, our thoughts and emotions are like clouds in the sky. Sometimes the sky is full of clouds. Those clouds may be white, grey or black. They may be low or high. They may be thick or thin. They may even be filled with thunder, lightning and torrential rain. At other times, the sky is cloudless and filled with sunlight. Clouds come and go. No matter how many or what kind of clouds there are, they never harm, touch, sully or diminish the essential nature of the space within which they move.

Based on this analogy, it makes little sense to battle with our thoughts and emotions. They come unbidden and they depart without our leave. Positive thoughts and pleasurable emotions may be replaced by negative thoughts and painful feelings, but none of these remains for ever and none of them ever touches or stains our essential nature. Therefore, when we are overwhelmed with negative emotions, guilt, self-loathing, fear and doubt, it is best if we simply acknowledge these feelings and let them be. The more we comment on them and try to push them about, the more we perpetuate them. Instead, if we simply note their arising, relax our muscular tension and keep breathing, we will find that, like dew on the morning grass, they have soon disappeared. So it is best to let your thoughts and emotions be, like clouds in the sky, and realise that ultimately they do not, cannot, touch us.

FINDING PURPOSE AND MEANING IN YOUR LIFE

It is widely believed in Asia that true happiness comes from doing what needs to be done despite how you may feel about it at the moment. Finding a purpose and meaning in life can be extremely helpful to anyone experiencing depression. Naturally, getting up and doing something, even something useful and important, seems impossible in the midst of a depressive episode when you are feeling hopeless and helpless and have lost all sense of meaning and direction. Once you have overcome the initial phase of a depressive episode, you will, all being well, find the strength and inspiration to continue. Finding such purpose and meaning through social, political, ecological, artistic or spiritual activities can help overcome momentary setbacks and temporary negative feelings. If you are focused on a goal that is larger than you, it is easier to rise to the occasion and, like an elephant walking through the jungle, plod forward step by step no matter what is in front of you. Meaningful activity is the root of self-esteem and doing what needs to be done next is a sure route to success.

A WORD ABOUT COMBINING PSYCHOTHERAPY WITH CHINESE MEDICINE

In cases where a long history of psychological trauma underlies a tendency towards depression, we do recommend that acupuncture and Chinese medicine be combined with psychotherapy by a qualified therapist. Psychotherapy and counselling can help speed the healing process as well as identify and effectively deal with any crises, such as thoughts of suicide.

In our experience, acupuncture not only assists the process of psychotherapy but can also enhance the depth and scope of therapy and help expedite progress. Many people who have repeatedly worked on their issues in therapy make a forward leap in that therapy when they start acupuncture treatment.

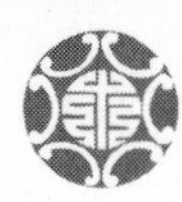

KICKING THE ANTIDEPRESSANT HABIT

Some of you may be currently using Western antidepressants. Do not discontinue medication abruptly without first checking with your doctor for advice on how best to reduce medication.

The ideal situation is where your doctor and practitioner of Chinese medicine work can work hand in hand. Do keep your practitioner informed as to medication. Generally speaking, Chinese medicine complements Western medicine very well. You may find that your Western medication is more effective and you suffer fewer side-effects if you are also being treated with Chinese medicine. Chinese medicine can be helpful and supportive if you are trying to reduce your medication and can lessen withdrawal symptoms, as well as helping to deal with the illness itself.

Anyone who may be suffering from severe mental problems, such as schizophrenia or bipolar disorder (manic depressive disorder), should not stop taking their Western medication. Chinese medicine may be supportive, or help to relieve unwanted side-effects from Western medication, but it is not sufficient as the only therapy or treatment for these conditions. If there is any risk of suicide or the depressive episode is severe, then we recommend that you immediately seek help from a doctor and or psychotherapist.

A CONTROLLED STUDY OF ACUPUNCTURE IN THE TREATMENT OF DEPRESSION

In 1993, the Office of Alternative Medicine (OAM) of the National Institutes of Health (NIH) in America funded 30 exploratory grants to encourage collaboration between conventional researchers and practitioners of alternative medicine. The purpose of these grants was to conduct small-scale preliminary studies to investigate whether some alternative therapies might warrant further study in the treatment of certain conditions.

In collaboration with John J.B. Allen, PhD, a professor of clinical psychology at the University of Arizona in Tucson, one of the authors of this book designed a study of acupuncture in the treatment of depression in women. The aim of our study was not only to determine the efficacy of acupuncture in treating depression but also to explore Chinese medicine's individual treatment approach within the framework of established scientific research protocols. We were fortunate to be one of the 30 studies initially funded by the OAM and one of only two to study acupuncture.

Because the size of these grants was very small compared to typical grants made by the NIH for 'conventional' medical research, we were forced to narrow our focus to a particular group of patients within the larger population of all possible sufferers of depression. This group was made up of women 18–45 years of age. However, based on our clinical experience and supported by statistical data, it is members of this group who suffer most commonly from depression.

DESCRIPTION OF THE STUDY

Altogether, 38 women aged 18–45 were recruited through newspaper advertisements. These advertisements offered 'non-drug' treatment for depression but did not mention acupuncture. The participants were first interviewed over the phone to see if they met our exclusion criteria. Women suffering from dysthymia, chronic depression, bipolar disorder, a history of psychosis or mania or other current clinical psychiatric disorders were excluded, as were women with substance abuse or dependency within the past four months who were undergoing current treatment for depression (psychotherapy or pharmacotherapy). Women who had endocrine abnormalities (thyroid disorder, Addison's diseases, etc.), lesions of the central nervous system, seizure disorders and pregnant women were also excluded. Women who presented with an active potential for suicide were excluded as well.

Study design

After the phone interview, those women who met the criteria for the study received a Structural Clinical Interview (SCID). This is a standard psychological interview to determine if they meet the DSM-IV criteria for major depression (Diagnostic and Statistical Manual of Mental Disorders, 4th edition). This interview was conducted by psychologists qualified to the level of a Master's degree.

A traditional Chinese medical diagnosis was then conducted by an acupuncturist to determine their Chinese pattern discrimination, treatment principles and acupuncture treatment plan. These treatments were designed by the assessing acupuncturist but were administered by four other acupuncturists. Neither the assessing acupuncturist nor the treating acupuncturists knew which treatment group the patient was in.

Participants were assigned to one of three groups: specific, non-specific and wait-list. Patients assigned to the specific group each received acupuncture treatment specifically to treat depression. Patients assigned to the non-specific group received treatment which was aimed at their Chinese pattern of disharmony but which did not address depression directly. Patients assigned to the wait-list group waited before receiving specific treatment. All treatments were tailored to the individual and were based on Chinese medical pattern discrimination.

The specific group received eight weeks of specific treatment. The non-specific group received eight weeks of non-specific treatment and then eight weeks of specific treatment. The wait-list group waited eight weeks and then received eight weeks of specific treatment. Each eight-week segment consisted of 12 sessions: two sessions per week for four weeks, then one session per week for four more weeks. By the end of this study, all participants had received specific treatment to address their pattern of disharmony as it related to their depression.

In addition to the SCID interview at the beginning of the study, participants were also assessed on the Hamilton Rating Scale for Depression (HRSD) before treatment began and again after four and eight weeks in the specific treatment group. In addition the non-specific and wait-list treatment groups were reassessed after 12 and 16 weeks. Patients also filled out self-report forms. Alliance to the therapist and resistance to treatment were also measured.

Study results

After completion of the specific treatment, using the DSM-IV remission criteria, 64 per cent of the women experienced full remission, 18 per cent of the women experienced partial remission and 18 per cent experienced no remission. Using the HRSD as the criterion for remission, 70 per cent of all women experienced remission, while 30 per cent did not.

These results compare favourably with both psychotherapy and pharmacotherapy whose effectiveness falls between 65–70 per cent. The drop-out rate was only 13 per cent in the acupuncture study, compared to over 30 per cent in most other studies. Specific acupuncture treatment produced a significant reduction of symptoms over time and it demonstrated greater reduction in symptoms over eight weeks than the non-specific group. However, it did not demonstrate a significantly greater reduction than the wait-list group.

Conclusions

These preliminary findings suggest that acupuncture is as effective as pharmacotherapy or psychotherapy as a treatment for depression. In addition, this study is a first attempt at conducting research according to established research protocols while respecting the individualised nature of Chinese medicine. It indicates that people who suffer from depression benefit from acupuncture treatment per se and not just because they expect to get better or because they derive benefit from interacting with a therapist.

WHAT DOES THIS RESEARCH MEAN FOR SUFFERERS OF DEPRESSION?

Due to the limited nature of the study, the sample of women included was very small. Therefore, these findings are clearly preliminary. A larger-scale study with many more women corroborating our findings will be necessary before acupuncture will be recognised as a viable treatment for depression by the scientific community. Nevertheless, this study does suggest that acupuncture is just as effective for the treatment of depression as psychotherapy and drug therapy. Since acupuncture as a part of Chinese medicine seeks to rebalance the health of the entire organism, body and mind, we feel that the total healing impact of this treatment is greater than that of either psychotherapy or drug therapy alone. In addition, professionally administered acupuncture has no or extremely minimal side-effects (occasional black and blue marks). Therefore, we think that people suffering from depression should consider acupuncture and Chinese medicine as either an alternative or complement to conventional Western therapy.

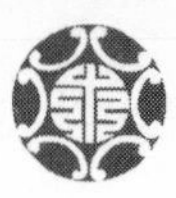

MORE CASE HISTORIES

In order to help readers get a better feel for how Chinese medicine treats depression, we have included some more case histories. We hope that these stories will encourage you to try acupuncture and Chinese medicine for yourself.

ADRIANNA

Adrianna was 27 years old. When she sought treatment with Chinese medicine she was currently on medication for depression and anxiety. She wanted to start a family and didn't want to continue on medication. She had been told by her doctor that, given her tendency towards recurrent depression and her family history of depression, she needed to stay on antidepressants for the rest of her life. She was determined to find an alternative.

At the onset of the latest episode, Adrianna had been under a lot of stress due to numerous life changes. She felt lethargic, had trouble concentrating, felt withdrawn and couldn't interact socially. She felt emotionally and physically drained and cried constantly. Her appetite was erratic, she felt bloated, was nauseous and experienced diarrhoea during stressful events. She felt tired all the time, yet she couldn't sleep well, waking up regularly through the night. Her thoughts raced constantly and she felt anxious and restless.

Adrianna had been on birth control pills for five years and had just stopped taking them a few months after the onset of her depression. She had a history of long cycles, inconsistent, dark menstrual flow and cramping both at ovulation and during her period. Premenstrually, she experienced abdominal bloating, breast distension, lower backache, leg pain, acne on her face, upper back and chest areas and a worsening of her depressive symptoms. She had not had a period for several months.

On examination, Adrianna's tongue was very puffy but dark and had a thin, frothy, white coating, especially on the sides. Her pulse was bowstring and a bit rapid but very deep and weak in the third or proximal positions on both sides.

Adrianna's Chinese medical pattern discrimination was read as liver depression qi stagnation and slight depressive heat affecting the heart with underlying spleen qi vacuity, damp accumulation and possibly kidney vacuity. Therefore the treatment principles were to course the liver and rectify the qi, clear heat and resolve depression while fortifying the spleen and transforming dampness. If, as treatment progressed, kidney yang vacuity became more evident, it would be addressed accordingly. Because her period had not come for several months and because of some of her specific menstrual symptoms, the principles of quickening the blood and regulating the menses were added to her treatment plan. Adrianna was given the following Chinese medical prescription:

9 g Radix Bupleuri *(Chai Hu)*
9 g Radix Scutellariae Baicalensis *(Huang Qin)*
9 g Radix Panacis Ginseng *(Ren Shen)*
4.5 g Rhizoma Pinelliae Ternatae *(Ban Xia)*
4.5 g Mix-fried Radix Glycyrrhizae *(Gan Cao)*
3 g Uncooked Rhizoma Zingiberis *(Sheng Jiang)*
4.5 g Radix Angelicae Sinensis *(Dang Gui)*
9 g Radix Ligustici Wallichii *(Chuang Xiong)*
9 g Rhizoma Cyperi Rotundi *(Xiang Fu)*
6 g Sclerotium Poriae Cocos *(Fu Ling)*
6 g Radix Polygalae Tenuifoliae *(Yuan Zhi)*
6 g Semen Zizyphi Spinosae *(Suan Zao Ren)*

The above Chinese medicinals were decocted in water and administered in two divided doses per day after breakfast and lunch. In addition, Adrianna received regular acupuncture sessions once a week. Some of the points used in her acupuncture sessions were:

Tai Chong (Liver 3)
He Gu (Large intestine 4)
Zhong Wan (Conception vessel 12)
Gong Sun (Spleen 4)
Nei Guan (Pericardium 6)
San Yin Jiao (Spleen 6)

She was able to decrease her medication gradually, both the antidepressant and the medication for anxiety, until she was able to discontinue them completely. After taking the decoction for three weeks, she continued with the acupuncture sessions for several more weeks, tapering off to maintenance treatments once a month. Adrianna was instructed to diminish her consumption of wheat and dairy products, eliminate sweets from her diet and exercise regularly, as well as to develop a relaxation routine. She no longer feels depressed, sleeps soundly through the night and is preparing to start a family. Adrianna's cycles have become more regular and she has experienced a decrease of premenstrual symptoms.

ELANA

Elana was 47 years old. She had experienced the loss of three very significant people in her life in the past several months. She had been clinically diagnosed with depression two weeks prior to her first visit. Upon questioning, it appeared that she had experienced severe depressive episodes a few times in the course of her life. She was now on an antidepressant but was experiencing uncomfortable side-effects and still felt depressed. She had nightmares and crying spells, felt hopeless and was very sad most of the time. Her appetite was erratic, she burped constantly, she was constipated and she had a history of gastric ulcers. Elana felt irritable and extremely anxious. She couldn't calm herself down and periodically erupted angrily at the people around her. She still had regular periods. However, these were becoming shorter in duration, scantier in amount and were a bit clotted. She had no significant premenstrual symptoms. Her pulse was slippery, rapid and bowstring on both sides. Her tongue was swollen and reddish with a thick, yellowish-white coating. Elana's Chinese medical pattern differentiation was read as phlegm heat internally harassing with concomitant liver depression. The Chinese medicinal prescription recommended for her was composed of:

9 g Rhizoma Pinelliae Ternatae *(Ban Xia)*
9 g Sclerotium Poriae Cocos *(Fu Ling)*
4.5 g Mix-fried Radix Glycyrrhizae *(Gan Cao)*
9 g Pericarpium Citri Reticulatae (*Chen Pi)*
3 g Uncooked Rhizoma Zingiberis *(Sheng Jiang)*
9 g Caulis Bambusae In Taeniis *(Zhu Ru)*
9 g Fructus Immaturus Citri Aurantii *(Zhi Shi)*
3 g Fructus Zizyphi Jujubae *(Da Zao)*
3 g Rhizoma Coptis Chinensis *(Huan Lian)*
4.5 g Semen Ziziyphi Spinosae *(Suan Zao Ren)*
4.5 g Rhizoma Acori Graminei *(Shi Chang Pu)*
6 g Radix Salviae Miltiorrhizae *(Dan Shen)*
4.5 g Tuber Curcumae *(Yu Jin)*
4.5 g Radix Polygalae Tenuifoliae *(Yuan Zhi)*

Elana discontinued the antidepressants and took the ingredients of this formula for two weeks in decoction form. Then, due to travelling and her busy schedule, she discontinued the decoction but continued on two formulae in tablet form, which combined most of the above mentioned ingredients. She called the office several weeks later to ask for a new supply of the tablets and reported she was feeling very well. She no longer felt depressed, she was sleeping well and she no longer felt irritable and anxious. In addition, all her digestive problems had completely disappeared.

ROBERT

Robert was 52 years old. He was feeling extremely hopeless and sad. He was very critical of himself and had a very poor self-image. He felt exhausted at the end of the day and had difficulty catching up after a long day of work. He also cried easily. Because this was extremely embarrassing in front of his friends, he had become isolated. All these conditions had become more evident in the last couple of years after a long-term relationship had ended. Robert had been on antidepressants briefly a few months previously, but he didn't want to go back on medication. He felt nauseous a lot, had no appetite and described a sinking feeling in his chest. This was accompanied by breathlessness, sighing and a sensation of something stuck in his throat. He experienced frequent night-time urination and had lower backache. His tongue was very swollen and pale with a slight purplish tinge and a wet, thin, white coating. Robert's pulse was slightly slippery but mostly weak and empty.

The reading of Robert's Chinese medical pattern differentiation was spleen–kidney yang vacuity giving rise to phlegm dampness obstruction and stagnation. Therefore, the treatment principles were to fortify the spleen and invigorate the kidneys, downbear counterflow and transform phlegm. Based on these principles, Robert was given a decoction which included the following ingredients:

12 g Rhizoma Pinelliae Ternata *(Ban Xia)*
9 g Cortex Magnoliae Officinalis *(Huo Po)*
6 g Folium Perillae Frutescentis *(Zi Su Ye)*
9 g Sclerotium Poriae Cocos *(Fu Ling)*
4.5 g Fructus Zizyphi Jujubae *(Da Zao)*
3 g Uncooked Rhizoma Zingiberis *(Sheng Jiang)*
9 g Radix Panacis Ginseng *(Ren Shen)*
6 g Rhizoma Atractylodis Macrocephalae *(Bai Zhu)*
4.5 g Cortex Cinnamomi Cassiae *(Rou Gui)*
6 g Cortex Eucommiae Ulmoidis *(Du Zhong)*

6 g Semen Cuscutae Chinensis *(Tu Si Zi)*
4.5 g Radix Bupleuri *(Chai Hu)*
4.5 g Pericarpium Citri Reticulatae Viride *(Qing Pi)*

Robert took the prescription above as a decoction twice per day. In addition, he was instructed to limit his intake of uncooked foods and cold drinks and to begin a sensitive exercise programme. He also received five acupuncture sessions, which consisted of stimulating the following points with needles:

Pi Shu (Bladder 20)
Shen Shu (Bladder 23)
Feng Long (Stomach 40)
Lie Que (Lung 7)
Dan Zhong (Conception vessel 17)
Nei Guan (Pericardium 6)
Tai Chong (Liver 3)
Tai Xi (Kidney 3)

After beginning the above treatments, Robert reported feeling much more energetic and enthusiastic. He began doing voluntary work at his local community centre. His appetite improved, he no longer needed to urinate at night and his back didn't hurt as often.

CARMEN

Carmen was 35 years old. She had experienced low-grade depression for as long as she could remember. Lately, she felt stuck, had no interest in anything and was having a lot of difficulty making decisions. She felt guilty a lot of the time and alternated between being extremely fatigued and overly irritable. Carmen said that she had always felt like an outsider in her own world. She had a history of chronic constipation, her appetite was not very good, her hair was limp, her skin and lips were very dry and she experienced heart palpitations. Her menstrual cycles were long and her periods were scanty, a bit dark and clotted. Premenstrually, she had sharp breast pain, increased irritability and difficulty falling asleep. Her tongue was puffy and pale but darker on the sides and tip. Her pulse was bowstring and very fine.

Carmen's Chinese medical pattern differentiation was liver depression qi stagnation with blood vacuity. The treatment principles were to course the liver and rectify the qi, nourish the liver and supplement the blood. Carmen was given a decoction which consisted of the following ingredients:

7.5 g Radix Bupleuri *(Chai Hu)*
9 g Radix Angelicae Sinensis *(Dang Gui)*
9 g Radix Albus Paeoniae Lactiflorae *(Bai Shao)*
6 g Rhizoma Atractylodis Macrocephalae *(Bai Zhu)*
6 g Sclerotium Poriae Cocos *(Fu Ling)*
4.5 g Mix-fried Radix Glycyrrhizae *(Gan Cao)*
3 g Herba Menthae Haplocalycis *(Bo He)*
3 g Uncooked Rhizoma Zingiberis *(Sheng Jiang)*
6 g Fructus Lycii Chinensis *(Gou Ci Zi)*
4.5 g Semen Biotae Orientalis *(Bai Zi Ren)*
4.5 g Cortex Albizziae Julibrissinis *(He Huan Pi)*

In addition, Carmen was instructed to include a bit more animal protein in her diet, while minimising uncooked and chilled foods. After taking the decoction for four weeks, Carmen's cycle was not long as it had been. Instead, it came precisely at 28 days. She experienced very little premenstrual discomfort, was able to fall asleep easily and had no breast pain. In addition, Carmen gained enough confidence to change jobs and terminate a relationship that was no longer nurturing to her.

ALAN

Alan was 45 years old and was an important executive of a large firm. He had always been able to work hard and for long hours, and to meet deadlines. Alan was proud of making personal sacrifices for the success of his company. Lately, however, he had been extremely hostile towards his co-workers. He became annoyed and frustrated easily. Further, Alan said he had lost interest in his job, had no contact with his friends and had withdrawn from his family. After working 12–15 hours a day, he drank heavily and collapsed at the weekend. He felt a feeling of tightness and oppression in his chest, sighed frequently and felt tired all the time. He often woke in the middle of the night with nightmares. People close to Alan had made repeated suggestions about his condition, but he was unwilling to consider changing his patterns. After nearly being involved in a head-on traffic collision, Alan decided he needed to do something. His wife suggested he try acupuncture.

When Alan came in for his first visit, his tongue was dark and reddish and had a frothy, white coating on the centre towards the sides. His pulse was extremely bowstring and rapid. Based on these signs and all the symptoms he reported above, Alan's Chinese medical pattern discrimination was liver depression qi stagnation which had progressed into depressed and bound heat, dampness and blood. The treatment principles, therefore, were to course the liver and rectify the qi, clear heat and resolve depression, transform dampness and quicken the blood. Based on these principles, the Chinese medicinal formula chosen for Alan was composed of the following ingredients:

9 g Rhizoma Cyperi Rotundi *(Xiang Fu)*
6 g Radix Ligustici Wallichii *(Chiang Xiong)*
6 g Fructus Gardeniae Jasminoidis *(Zhi Zi)*
6 g Rhizoma Atractylodis *(Cang Zhu)*
4.5 g Massa Medica Fermentata *(Shen Qu)*

4.5 g Rhizoma Acori Graminei *(Shi Chang Pu)*
4.5 g Tuber Curcumae *(Yu Jin)*
3 g Rhizoma Coptidis Chinensis *(Huan Lian)*

In addition, Alan received eight acupuncture sessions, which consisted of some of the following points:

Xiang Jian (Liver 2)
Tai Chong (Liver 3)
He Gu (Large intestine 4)
Qu Chi (Large intestine 11)
Da Ling (Pericardium 7)
Qi Men (Liver 14)
Jiu Wei (Conception vessel 15)
Yin Tang[7]

Alan reported that he felt calmer, more even-tempered and more enthusiastic about his job. He decided to do some short-term cognitive therapy to help him develop strategies to cope better with stress and to balance work with personal interests and family life. He continued bi-monthy acupuncture sessions for about six months, and at the same time developed exercise and relaxation routines and continued trying to limit his time at the office. He no longer feels tightness and oppression in his chest, he sleeps well most of the time and he drinks only occasionally at social events.

CONCLUSIONS

As the above case histories show, Chinese medicine treats the whole person. It is not just symptomatic treatment. In all cases, the patients not only overcame their depression, but other of their symptoms also 'miraculously' disappeared. Actually, there is nothing miraculous about this. If these

---

[7] Yin Tang is an extra point and is not located on one of the main channels.

accompanying symptoms had not disappeared, the Chinese doctor would have thought that the treatment was not completely successful.

Although Chinese medicine does not work immediately, because it treats the whole person, it is usually worth waiting and persevering. Western antidepressants also take some time to begin acting, but they also usually produce unpleasant side-effects. In addition, once people understand that Chinese medicine is not a symptomatic 'quick fix', they are motivated to keep on with a good diet, regular exercise and daily deep relaxation.

FINDING A PROFESSIONAL PRACTITIONER OF CHINESE MEDICINE

Chinese medicine has grown enormously in the UK during the past 30 years. There are at least 10 colleges that offer professional training, some offering a university degree.

Many excellent practitioners have come to the UK from China, Vietnam and other countries of East Asia.

As you will no doubt have realised after reading this book, Chinese medicine is a whole system of medicine with its own fundamental concepts and theories. It is not simply a technique. Previous knowledge or training in another system of medicine does not automatically confer competence or knowledge in Chinese medicine. In order to get the most out of your therapy or treatment you should ensure that the practitioner is properly qualified. Currently in the UK the onus is on the individual to check the qualifications and training of their practitioner. In order to help you to do this we have listed the relevant professional bodies covering Chinese medicine. Members of these professional organisations are bound by a professional code of ethics and practice. They will have received an accredited level of training and will be covered by medical malpractice and public/products liability insurance.

When trying to find a good practitioner one of the best methods is by personal recommendation. It is also important that you are able to communicate with the practitioner should English not be their first language. It is quite acceptable to ask about their previous experience in treating your complaint. Many practitioners will be happy to talk on the phone or may offer a short introductory consultation so that you can assess whether you will feel comfortable working with them.

In addition to Chinese, I have included Japanese traditions of herbal medicine (kanpo) and massage (shiatsu). They originate from the same basic sources but have evolved differently in terms of style and practice.

The relevant professional bodies for Chinese medicine in the UK are:

Acupuncture
The British Acupuncture Council
63 Jeddo Road
London
W12 9HQ
Tel: 020 8735 0400
Fax: 020 8735 0404
E-mail: infor@acupuncture.org.uk
Website: www.acupuncture.org.uk

Members have the initials: MBAcC.

Chinese herbal medicine
The Register of Chinese Herbal Medicine
PO Box 400
Wembley
Middlesex
HA9 9NZ
Tel/fax: 07000 790332
Website: www.rchm.co.uk

Members have the initials: MRCHM.

Japanese herbal medicine
The Kanpo Association
9a Ingatestone Road
Brentwood
Essex
CM15 8AP
Tel: 01277 260080

Members have the initials: KANPO.
Members of the Kanpo Association are not bound by a code of ethics and practice or covered by insurance unless they also belong to another professional body. Most practitioners of kanpo belong to one of the three other professional bodies.

Shiatsu
The Shiatsu Society UK
Barber House
Storeys Bar Road
Fengate
Peterborough
PE1 5YS
Tel: 01733 758341
E-mail: shiatsu@graphic-scan.co.uk

Members have the initials: MRSS.

Relevant bodies in other English-speaking countries are:

Australian Acupuncture and Chinese Medical Association
PO Box 5142
West End
Brisbane
Queensland
Australia 4101
Tel: +07 3846 5866
Fax: +07 3846 5276
Free Call: 1800 025 334
E-mail: aaca@eis.net.all
Website: http://www2.eis.net.au/-aaca

AACMA is apparently the best professional organisation within Australia for patient contact.

The International Institute of Chinese Medicine and Acupuncture
PO Box 2246
19 Av Disandt-Fresnaye
Cape Town 8000
South Africa
Tel: 27 21 434 1654

LEARNING MORE ABOUT CHINESE MEDICINE

Acupuncture and Chinese medicine in general

Chinese Medicine: Acupuncture, Herbal Remedies, Nutrition, Qui Gong and Meditation, Tom Williams, Element Health Essentials
This is a good basic introduction to the whole field of Chinese medicine for the layperson.

Acupuncture, Peter Mole, Element Books
A simple and clear introduction to acunpuncture fo the layperson.

A Guide to Acupuncture, Peter Firebrace and Sandra Hill, Constable Books
A comprehensive introduction to acupuncture for the layperson with some illustrations and photographs.

Between Heaven and Earth: A Guide to Chinese Medicine, Harriet Beinfield and Efrem Corngold, Ballantine Books, New York
This book is particularly good with regard to the more psychological and emotional aspects of Chinese medicine and has a good introduction to herbal medicine for the layperson.

Acupuncture in Practice, Hugh McPherson and Ted Kaptchuk (eds), Churchill Livingston
This is a book of case histories from the West; it illustrates the wide variety of styles and methods of practice of acupuncture by many well-known practitioners.

Chinese Herbal Medicine, a Practical Guide to the Healing Powers of Herbs, Dr Guang Xu, Vermillion
A good introduction to Chinese herbal medicine.

*Japanese Acupuncture, a Clinical Guid*e, Stephen Birch and Junko Ida, Paradigm Publications
This book gives very good, clear details on moxibustion.

Chinese dietary therapy

Healing with Wholefoods, Oriental Traditions and Modern Nutrition, Paul Pritchard, North Atlantic Books
A comprehensive source book for both the layperson and the professional.

Helping Ourselves: A Guide to the Traditional Chinese Food Energetics, Daverick Legget, Meridian Press
This book is designed for ease of use with its clear layout and wallcharts.

Chinese Medical Wines and Elixirs, Bob Flaws, Blue Poppy Press, Boulder, Colorado.

The Book of Jook: Chinese Medical Porridges: A Healthy Alternative to the Typical Western Breakfast, Bob Flaws, Blue Poppy Press, Boulder, Colorado.

Chinese Medicinal Teas: Simple, Proven, Folk Formulas for Common Diseases and Promoting Health, Zong Xiao-fan and Gary Liscum, Blue Poppy Press, Boulder, Colorado.

SUPPLIERS OF CHINESE MEDICINES

Acumedic
101–5 Camden High Street
London
NW1 7JN
Tel: 0171 388 5783
Fax: 0171 387 5766

Beijing Tong Ren Tang
124 Shaftesbury Avenue
London
W1V 7DJ
Tel: 0171 287 0098
Fax: 0171 287 0068

China Medica
25 Lonsdale Close
London
SE9 4HF
Tel: 0181 857 9777
Fax: 0181 480 2020

Chinese Medical Centre
179 South Street
Romford
Essex
RM1 1PS
Tel: 01708 756363
Fax: 01708 703015

East West Herbs
Langston Priory Mews
Kingham
Oxfordshire
OX7 6UP
Tel: 01608 658862
Fax: 01608 658816
E-mail: robert@eastwestherbs.co.uk

Great Wall
Unit 27
Riverside Works
Hertford Road
Barking
Essex
IG11 8BN
Tel: 0181 591 6896
Fax: 0181 591 6891

Harmony Medical Distribution
629 High Road
Leytonstone
London
E11 4PA
Tel: 0181 518 7337
Fax: 0181 556 5038
E-mail: harmony@tcm.org.uk

Lotus
Priorsfield Priory
Forest Row
Sussex
RH18 5HR
Tel: 01342 823053
Fax: 01342 826027
E-mail: user@lotus.u-net.com

Mayway UK
43 Waterside Trading Centre
Trumpers Way
Hanwell
Middlesex
Tel: 0181 893 6873
Fax: 0181 893 6874

Naturally Chinese
P.O. Box 4584
Kiln Farm
Milton Keynes
Bucks
MK13 9BT
Tel: 0151 571 0407

Number One Herb Co
36 Bankhurst Road
Catford
London
SE6 4XN
Tel: 0181 690 4840
Fax: 0181 690 4840
E-mail: jarrah@vossnet.co.uk

Oxford Medical Supplies
Units 11 & 12
Horcott Industrial Estate
Fairford
Gloucestershire
GL7 4LX
Tel: 0800 975 8000
Fax: 0800 975 8111
E-mail: oxfordms@demon.co.uk

Shizhen TCM UK Ltd
50 Sandy Lane
Chorlton
Manchester
M21
Tel: 0161 881 0088
Fax: 0161 881 0888

Tian Tiao Ltd
85 Sullivan Way
Elstree
Herts
WD6 3DG
Tel: 0181 953 2320
Fax: 0181 953 3338

CHINESE MEDICAL GLOSSARY

Chinese medicine is a system unto itself. Its technical terms are uniquely its own and cannot be reduced to the definitions of Western medicine without destroying the very fabric and logic of Chinese medicine. Ultimately, because Chinese medicine was created in the Chinese language, Chinese medicine is really only understood in that language. Nevertheless, as Westerners trying to understand Chinese medicine, we must translate the technical terms of Chinese medicine in English words. If some of these technical translations sound peculiar at first and their meaning is not immediately clear, this is because no equivalent concepts exist in everyday English.

In the past, some Western authors have erroneously translated technical Chinese medical terms using Western medical or at least quasi-scientific words in an attempt to make this system more acceptable to Western audiences. For instance, the words 'tonify' and 'sedate' are commonly seen in the Western Chinese medical literature even though, in the case of 'sedate', its meaning is completely opposite to the Chinese understanding of the word *xie*. *Xie* means to drain off something that has pooled and accumulated. That accumulation is seen as something excess, which should not be lingering where it is. Because it is accumulating somewhere where it shouldn't, it is impeding and obstructing whatever should be moving to and through that area. The word 'sedate' comes from the Latin word *sedere*, to sit. Therefore, sedate means to make something sit still. However, the Chinese *xie* means draining off that which is sitting somewhere erroneously. Therefore, to think that one is going to sedate what is already sitting is a great mistake in understanding the clinical implication and application of this technical term.

Hence, in order to preserve the integrity of this system while still making it intelligible to English language readers, we have appended the following glossary of Chinese medical technical terms. The terms themselves are based on Nigel Wiseman's *English–Chinese Chinese–English Dictionary of Chinese Medicine* (see page 170). Dr Wiseman is, I believe, the greatest Western scholar in terms of the translation of Chinese medicine into English. Although Wiseman's terms may be awkward sounding at first, they convey most accurately the Chinese understanding and logic of these terms.

Acquired essence: Essence manufactured out of the surplus of qi and blood in turn created out of the refined essence of food and drink
Acupoints: Those places on the channels and network vessels where qi and blood tend to collect in denser concentrations and thus those places where the qi and blood in the channels are especially available for manipulation
Acupuncture: The regulation of qi flow by the stimulation of certain points located on the channels and network vessels achieved mainly by insertion of fine needles into these points
Astringent: Constricting and containing, keeping in rather than letting go
Bar: A position on the wrist where the pulse may be felt; *see* **Pulse**
Bedroom taxation: Fatigue or vacuity due to excessive sex
Blood: The red-coloured fluids that flow in the vessels and nourish and construct the tissues of the body
Blood stasis: Also called dead blood, malign blood and dry blood, blood stasis is blood that is no longer moving through the vessels as it should. Instead it is precipitated in the vessels like silt in a river. It obstructs the free flow of the blood in the vessels and also impedes the production of new or fresh blood
Blood vacuity: Insufficient blood manifesting in diminished nourishment, construction and moistening of body tissues

Bowels: The hollow yang organs of Chinese medicine
Bowstring: A quality of pulse that feels taut; *see* **Pulse**
Burners: Areas of the abdomen, known as the upper, middle and lower burners, that act as a kind of crucible in which the vital energies are transformed and created by heat
Central qi: Also called the middle qi, this is synonymous with the spleen–stomach qi
Channels: The main routes for the distribution of qi and blood, but mainly qi
Chest oppression: A feeling of tightness and stuffiness in the chest. As a reaction to this feeling, the person will often sigh in an attempt to inhale fresh air and exhale the pent-up stale air
Choppy: A choppy pulse is a fine, somewhat slow pulse which tends to speed up and slow down (often with the breathing) but does not necessarily skip any beats; *see* **Pulse**
Clear: The pure or clear part of ingested food and drink that is then turned into qi and blood
Constructive qi: The qi that flows through the channels and nourishes and constructs the internal organs and body tissues
Counterflow: An erroneous flow of qi, usually upwards but sometimes horizontally as well
Coursing the liver: Encouraging the correct functioning of the liver viscera with regard to the flow of qi throughout the body
Damp heat: A combination of accumulated dampness mixed with pathological heat often associated with sores, abnormal vaginal discharges and some types of menstrual and body pain
Dampness: A pathological accumulation of body fluids
Decoction: A method of administering Chinese medicinals by boiling these medicinals in water, straining off the dregs and drinking the resulting medicinal liquid
Deep: A pulse quality; *see* **Pulse**
Defensive qi: The yang qi that protects the exterior of the body from invasion by the environmental excesses
Depression: Stagnation and lack of movement, as in liver depression qi stagnation

Depressive heat: Heat due to enduring or severe qi stagnation, which then transforms into heat
Distal: A position where the pulse may be felt; *see* **Pulse**
Drain: To drain off or away some pathological qi or substance from where it is replete or excess
Empty pulse: A pulse quality; *see* **Pulse**
Environmental excesses: A superabundance of wind, cold, dampness, dryness, heat, or summer heat in the external environment that can invade the body and cause disease
Essence: A stored, very potent form of substance and qi, usually yin when compared to yang qi, but can be transformed into yang qi
External causes of disease: The six environmental excesses
Fine: A pulse quality; *see* **Pulse**
Fire (life gate fire, fire effulgence): A pathogenic factor that is usually created within the body
Five phase theory: An ancient Chinese system of correspondences dividing up all of reality into five phases, which then mutually engender and check each other according to definite sequences
Heart vexation: An irritating, possibly dry, hot sensation in the chest in front of the heart
Heat toxins: A particularly virulent and concentrated type of pathological heat often associated with purulence (i.e. pus formation), sores and sometimes, but not always, malignancies
Impediment: A hindrance to the free flow of the qi and blood typically manifesting as pain and restriction in the range of movement of a joint or extremity
Internal causes of disease: The seven effects or emotions, namely anger, joy (or excitement), sorrow, thought, fear, melancholy and fright
Lassitude of the spirit: A listless or apathetic effect or emotional demeanour due to obvious fatigue of the mind and body
Life gate fire: Another name for kidney yang or kidney fire,

seen as the ultimate source of yang qi in the body
Mansion: Realm of influence of one of the viscera
Moxibustion: Burning the herb Artemisia Argyium on, over or near acupuncture points in order to add yang qi, to warm cold, or promote the movement of the qi and blood
Neither external nor internal causes of disease: A miscellaneous group of pathogenic factors including trauma, diet, overtaxation, insufficient exercise, poisoning, parasites, etc.
Network vessels: Small vessels that form a net-like web insuring the flow of qi and blood to all body tissues
Pattern discrimination: Basis for diagnosis in TCM. A pattern is determined by the signs and symptoms and observations of the individual patient's condition
Phlegm: A pathological accumulation of phlegm or mucus congealed from dampness or body fluids
Portals: Also called orifices, the openings of the sensory organs and the opening of the heart through which the spirit makes contact with the world outside
Pulse: Taking the pulse forms an important part of Chinese medical diagnosis. It is taken from the radial artery at both wrists and there are six different pulse positions at each wrist, giving information about the different viscera, bowels and channels. There are 28 types of pulse quality in classic Chinese medicine, including deep, empty, fine, slippery, etc.
Qi: Activity, function, that which moves, transforms, defends, restrains and warms
Qi mechanism: The process of transforming yin substance controlled and promoted by the qi, largely synonymous with the process of digestion
Qi vacuity: Insufficient qi manifesting in diminished movement, transformation and function
Repletion: Excess or fullness, almost always pathological
Seven star hammer: A small hammer with needles embedded in its head used to stimulate acupoints without actually inserting needles

Slippery: A pulse quality; *see* **Pulse**
Soggy: A pulse quality; *see* **Pulse**
Spirit: The accumulation of qi in the heart that manifests as consciousness, sensory awareness and mental–emotional function
Stagnation: Non-movement of the qi, lack of free flow, constraint
Supplement: To add to or augment, as in supplementing the qi, blood, yin, or yang
Turbid: The yin, impure, turbid part of food and drink that is sent downwards to be excreted as waste
Vacuity: Emptiness or insufficiency, typically of qi, blood, yin, or yang
Vacuity cold: Obvious signs and symptoms of cold due to a lack or insufficiency of yang qi
Vacuity heat: Heat due to hyperactive yang in turn due to insufficient controlling yin
Vessels: The main routes for the distribution of qi and blood, but mainly blood
Viscera: The solid yin organs of Chinese medicine
Yang: In the body, function, movement, activity and transformation
Yang vacuity: Insufficient warming and transforming function giving rise to symptoms of cold in the body
Yin: In the body, substance and nourishment
Yin vacuity: Insufficient yin substance necessary to nourish, control and counterbalance yang activity

BIBLIOGRAPHY

CHINESE LANGUAGE SOURCES

Cheng Dan An Zhen Jiu Xuan Ji (Cheng Dan An's Selected Acupuncture and Moxibustion Works), Cheng Wei-fen *et al.* (eds), Shanghai Science and Technology Press, Shanghai, 1986

Chu Zhen Zhi Liao Xue (A Study of Acupuncture Treatment), Li Zhong-yu, Sichuan Science and Technology Press, Chengdu, 1990

Fu Ke Lin Chuan Jing Hua (The Clinical Efflorescence of Gynaecology), Wang Bu-ru and Wang Qi-ming, Sichuan Science and Technology Press, Chengdu, 1989

Fu Ke Yu Chi (The Jade Ruler of Gynaecology), Shen Jin-ao, Shanghai Science and Technology Press, Shanghai, 1983

Fu Ke Zheng Zhi (Gynaecological Patterns and Treatments), Sun Jiu-ling, Hebei People's Press, 1983

Gu Fang Miao Yong (Ancient Formulas, Wondrous Uses), Chen Bao-ming and Zhao Jin-xi, Science and Technology Popularization Press, Beijing, 1994

Han Ying Chang Yong Yi Xue Ci Hui (Chinese–English Glossary of Commonly Used Medical Terms), Huang Xiao-kai, People's Health and Hygiene Press, Beijing, 1982

Nan Zhi Bing De Liang Fang Miao Fa (Fine Formulas and Wondrous Methods for Difficult to Treat Diseases), Wu Da-zhen and He Xin-qiao, Chinese National Medicine and Medicinal Press, Beijing, 1992

Nei Ke Bing Liang Fang (Internal Medicine Disease Fine Formulas), He Yuan-lin and Jiang Chang-yuan, Yunnan University Press, Zhongqing, 1991

Qi Nan Za Zheng Jing (Carefully Chosen Curious, Difficult, Miscellaneous Diseases), Huang Bing-yuan, Guangdong Science and Technology Press, Guangzhou, 1996

'A Review of the Chinese Medical Literature on Climacteric

Syndrome', Yao Shi-an, *Zhong Yi Za Zhi (Journal of Chinese Medicine)*, No. 2, 1994
Shang Hai Lao Zhong Yi Jing Yan Xuan Bian (A Selected Compilation of Shanghai Old Doctors' Experiences), Shanghai Science and Technology Press, Shanghai, 1984
Shi Yong Zhen Jiu Tui Na Zhi Liao Xue (A Study of Practical Acupuncture, Moxibustion and Tui Na Treatments), Xia Zhi-ping, Shanghai College of Chinese Medicine Press, Shanghai, 1990
Tan Zheng Lun (Treatise on Phlegm Conditions), Hou Tian-yin and Wang Chun-hua, People's Army Press, Beijing, 1989
Xian Dai Nan Zhi Bing Zhong Yi Zhen Liao Xue (A Study of the Chinese Medical Diagnosis and Treatment of Modern Difficult to Treat Diseases), Wu Jun-yu and Bai Yong-bo, Chinese Medicine Ancient Books Press, Beijing, 1993
Yi Zong Jin Jian (The Golden Mirror of Ancestral Medicine), Wu Qian *et al.*, People's Health and Hygiene Press, Beijing, 1985
Yu Xue Zheng Zhi (Static Blood Patterns and Treatments), Zhang Xue-wen, Shanxi Science and Technology Press, Xian, 1986
Zhen Jiu Chu Fang Xue (A Study of Acupuncture and Moxibustion Prescriptions), Wang Dai, Beijing Publishing Co., Beijing, 1990
Zhen Jiu Da Cheng (A Great Compendium of Acupuncture and Moxibustion), Yang Ji-zhou, People's Health and Hygiene Press, Beijing, 1983
Zhen Jiu Xue (A Study of Acupuncture and Moxibustion), Qiu Mao-liang *et al.*, Shanghai Science and Technology Press, Shanghai, 1985
Zhen Jiu Yi Xue (An Easy Study of Acupuncture and Moxibustion), Li Shou-xian, People's Health and Hygiene Press, Beijing, 1990
Zhong Guo Min Jian Cao Yao Fang (Chinese Folk Herbal Medicinal Formulas), Liu Guang-rui and Liu Shao-lin, Sichuan Science and Technology Press, Chengdu, 1992
Zhong Guo Zhen Jiu Chu Fang Xue (A Study of Chinese

Acupuncture and Moxibustion Prescriptions), Xiao Shao-qing, Ningxia People's Press, Yinchuan, 1986

Zhong Guo Zhong Yi Mi Fang Da Quan (A Great Compendium of Chinese National Chinese Medical Secret Formulas), Hu Zhao-ming (ed.), Literary Propagation Publishing Company, Shanghai, 1992

Zhong Yi Bing Yin Bing Ji Xue (A Study of Chinese Medical Disease Causes and Disease Mechanisms), Wu Dun-xu, Shanghai College of Chinese Medicine Press, Shanghai, 1989

Zhong Yi Fu Ke Zhi Liao Shou Ce (A Handbook of Chinese Medical Gynaecological Treatment), Wu Shi-xing and Qi Cheng-lin, Shanxi Science and Technology Press, Xian, 1991

Zhong Yi Hu Li Xue (A Study of Chinese Medical Nursing), Lu Su-ying, People's Health and Hygiene Press, Beijing, 1983

Zhong Yi Lin Chuang Ge Ke (Various Clinical Specialties in Chinese Medicine), Zhang En-qin *et al.*, Shanghai College of TCM Press, Shanghai, 1990

Zhong Yi Ling Yan Fang (Efficacious Chinese Medical Formulas), Lin Bin-zhi, Science and Technology Propagation Press, Beijing, 1991

Zhong Yi Miao Yong Yu Yang Sheng (Chinese Medicine Wondrous Uses and Nourishing Life), Ni Qi-lan, Liberation Army Press, Beijing, 1993

Zhong Yi Nei Ke Lin Chuang Shou Ce (A Clinical Manual of Chinese Medicine Internal Medicine), Xia De-shu, Shanghai Science and Technology Press, Shanghai, 1990

Zhong Yi Nei Ke Xue (The Study of Chinese Internal Medicine), Zhang Bo-ying *et al.*, Shanghai Science and Technology Press, Shanghai, 1990

Zhong Yi Zi Xue Cong Shu (The Chinese Medicine Self-study Series), Vol. 1, 'Gynaecology', Yang Yi-ya, Hebei Science and Technology Press, Shijiazhuang, 1987

ENGLISH LANGUAGE SOURCES

Abnormal Psychology: Current Perspectives, B.L. Alloy, J. Acocella and R.R. Bootzin, McGraw Hill, New York, 1996

A Barefoot Doctor's Manual, revised and enlarged edition, Cloudburst Press, Mayne Isle, 1977

Beyond Prozac, Michael J. Norden, HarperCollins Publishers Inc., New York, 1995

Chinese–English Terminology of Traditional Chinese Medicine, Shuai Xue-zhong *et al.*, Hunan Science and Technology Press, Changsha, 1983

Chinese–English Manual of Common-used Prescriptions in Traditional Chinese Medicine, Ou Ming (ed.), Joint Publishing Co. Ltd, Hong Kong, 1989

Chinese Herbal Medicine: Formulas and Strategies, Dan Bensky and Randall Barolet, Eastland Press, Seattle, 1990

Chinese Herbal Medicine: Materia Medica, Dan Bensky and Andrew Gamble, second (revised) edition, Eastland Press, Seattle, 1993

Chinese Self-massage, The Easy Way to Health, Fan Ya-li, Blue Poppy Press, Boulder, Colorado, 1996

A Clinical Guide to Chinese Herbs and Formulae, Cheng Song-yu and Li Fei, Churchill and Livingstone, Edinburgh, 1993

A Clinical Manual of Chinese Herbal Medicine and Acupuncture, Zhou Zhong Ying and Jin Hui De, Churchill Livingstone, Edinburgh, 1997

A Compendium of TCM Patterns and Treatments, Bob Flaws and Daniel Finney, Blue Poppy Press, Boulder, Colorado, 1996

A Comprehensive Guide to Chinese Herbal Medicine, Chen Ze-lin and Chen Mei-fang, Oriental Healing Arts Institute, Long Beach, California, 1992

Diagnostic and Statistical Manual of Mental Disorders: Fourth Edition, American Psychiatric Association, Washington, DC, 1994

English–Chinese Chinese–English Dictionary of Chinese Medicine, Nigel Wiseman, Hunan Science and Technology

Press, Changsha, 1995
Fundamentals of Chinese Acupuncture, Andrew Ellis, Nigel Wiseman and Ken Boss, Paradigm Publications, Brookline, MA, 1988
Fundamentals of Chinese Medicine, Nigel Wiseman and Andrew Ellis, Paradigm Publications, Brookline, MA, 1985
Glossary of Chinese Medical Terms and Acupuncture Points, Nigel Wiseman and Ken Boss, Paradigm Publications, Brookline, MA, 1990
Handbook of Chinese Herbs and Formulas, Him-che Yeung, self-published, Los Angeles, 1985
A Handbook of Differential Diagnosis with Key Signs and Symptoms, Therapeutic Principles and Guiding Prescriptions, Ou-yang Yi, (trans. C.S. Cheung), Harmonious Sunshine Cultural Centre, San Francisco, 1987
A Handbook of Menstrual Diseases in Chinese Medicine, Bob Flaws, Blue Poppy Press, Boulder, Colorado, 1997
Oriental Materia Medica, A Concise Guide, Hong-yen Hsu, Oriental Healing Arts Institute, Long Beach, California, 1986
Practical Therapeutics of Traditional Chinese Medicine, Yan Wu and Warren Fischer, Paradigm Publications, Brookline, MA, 1997
Practical Traditional Chinese Medicine and Pharmacology: Clinical Experiences, Shang Xian-min *et al.*, New World Press, Beijing, 1990
Practical Traditional Chinese Medicine and Pharmacology: Herbal Formulas, Geng Jun-ying, *et al.*, New World Press, Beijing, 1991
Sacred Sorrow: Embracing and Transforming Depression, John E. Nelson and A. Nelson, Putnam and Sons Publishing, New York, 1996
The English–Chinese Encyclopaedia of Practical Traditional Chinese Medicine, Vol. 12: Gynaecology, Xuan Jia-sheng (ed.), Higher Education Press, Beijing, 1990

The Essential Book of Traditional Chinese Medicine, Vol. 2: Clinical Practice, Liu Yan-chi, (trans. Fang Ting-yu and Chen Lai-di), Columbia University Press, New York, 1988
The Foundations of Chinese Medicine, Giovanni Maciocia, Churchill Livingstone, Edinburgh, 1989
The Merck Manual, 15th edition, Robert Berkow (ed.), Merck Sharp and Dohme Research Laboratories, Rahway, New Jersey, 1987
The Nanjing Seminars Transcript, Qiu Mao-lian and Su Xu-ming, *The Journal of Chinese Medicine*, UK, 1985
The Practice of Chinese Medicine, Giovanni Maciocia, Churchill Livingstone, Edinburgh, 1994
'The Role of the Liver in Menstrual Disorders', (Rona) Wang Ru and Brian May, *The Pacific Journal of Oriental Medicine*, Australia, No. 77
'A Theoretical and Practical Approach to Psychodynamics Using Traditional Chinese Medicine', Daniel A. Weber, *The Pacific Journal of Oriental Medicine*, Mullimbimby, New South Wales, No. 10, 1997
The Treatise on the Spleen and Stomach, Li Dong-yuan, (trans. Yang Shou- zhong), Blue Poppy Press, Boulder, Colorado, 1993
The Treatment of Disease in TCM, Volume 1: Diseases of the Head and Face Including Mental/Emotional Disorders, Philippe Sionneau and Lu Gang, Blue Poppy Press, Boulder, Colorado, 1996
Traditional Medicine in Contemporary China, Nathan Sivin, University of Michigan, Ann Arbor, 1987
Zang Fu: The Organ Systems of Traditional Chinese Medicine (second edition), Jeremy Ross, Churchill Livingstone, Edinburgh, 1985.

INDEX

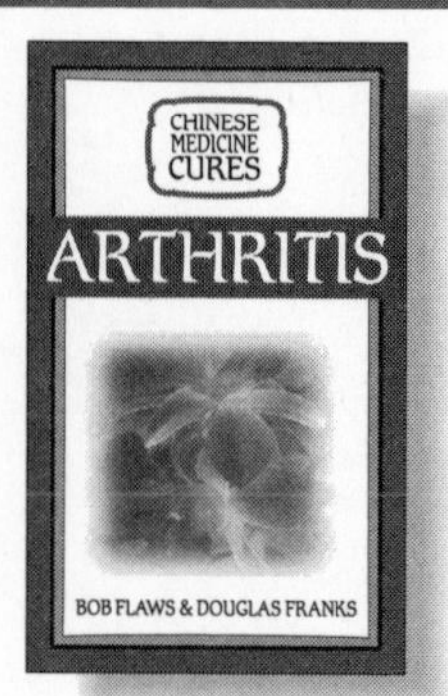

October 1999 -
Chinese Medicine Cures Arthritis -
ISBN: 0-572-02540-8

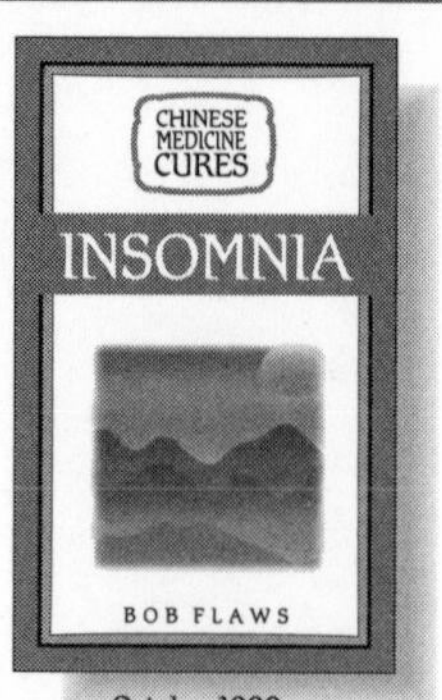

October 1999 -
Chinese Medicine Cures Insomnia -
ISBN: 0-572-02568-8

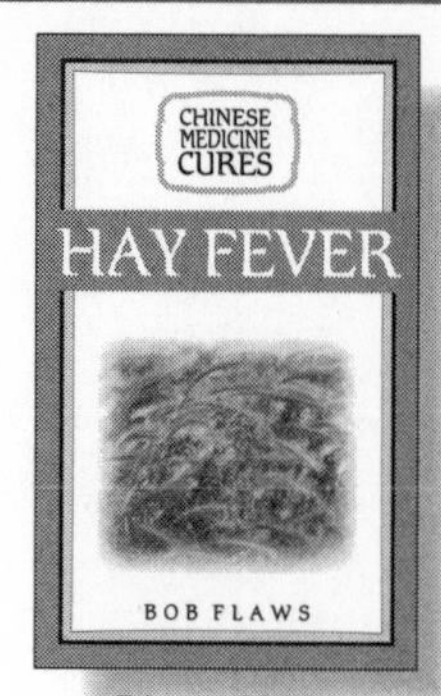

February 2000 -
Chinese Medicine Cures Hayfever -
ISBN: 0-572-02576-9

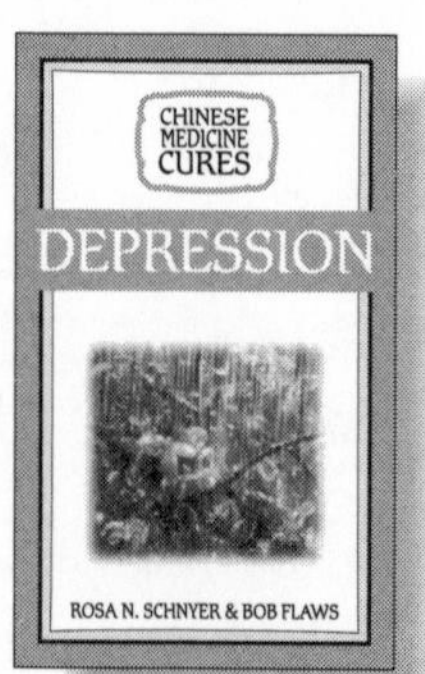

February 2000 -
Chinese Medicine Cures Depression -
ISBN: 0-572-02577-7

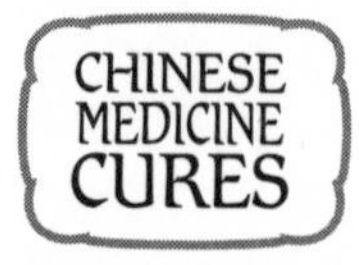

BY WORLD-RENOWNED EXPERT
BOB FLAWS
Governor of the National Academy of Acupuncture and Oriental Medicine
Fellow of The Register of Chinese Herbal Medicine.
Edited by
Sylvia Schroer BSc MRCHM MBAcC
Council Member of the Register of Chinese Medicine

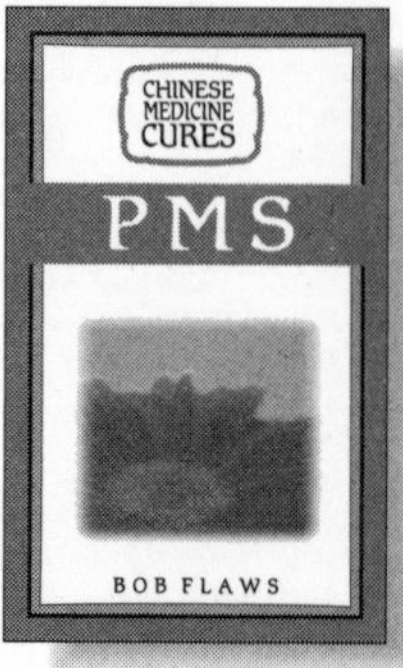

Summer 2000 -
Chinese Medicine Cures PMS - ISBN:
0-572-02539-4

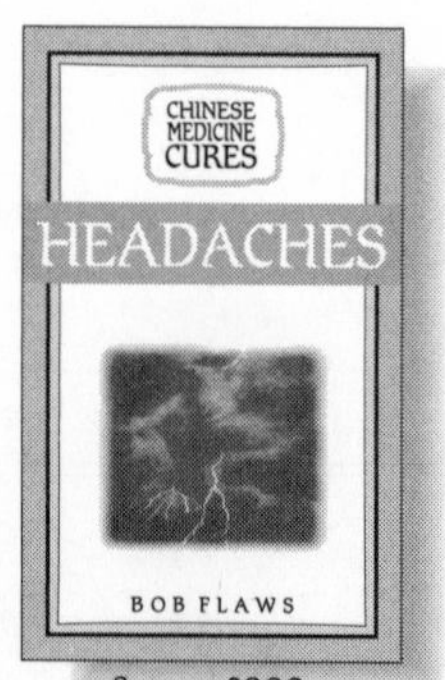

Summer 2000 -
Chinese Medicine Cures Headaches -
ISBN: 0-572-02590-4

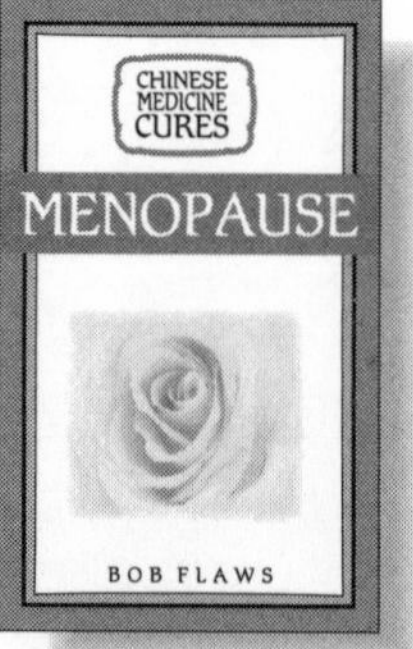

Autumn 2000 -
Chinese Medicine Cures Menopause -
ISBN: 0-572-02591-2

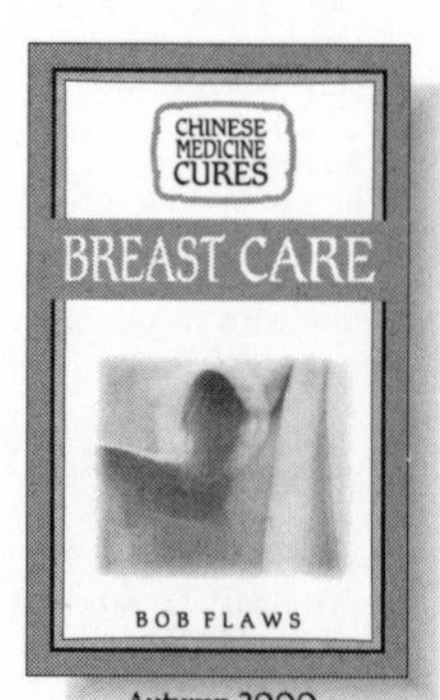

Autumn 2000 -
Chinese Medicine Cures Breast Care-
ISBN: 0-572-02592-0